SATAN'S SPAWN

Memories of a Medical man

G. W. Robinson

MINERVA PRESS
MONTREUX LONDON WASHINGTON

SATAN'S SPAWN

ISBN 1 85863 310 9

First Published 1994 by
MINERVA PRESS
10 Cromwell Place
London SW7 2JN

Printed in Great Britain by
B.W.D. Printers Ltd., Northolt, Middlesex

SATAN'S SPAWN

Memories of a Medical man

I was born on the 2nd September 1896. Naturally I have no memory of the event, but have to depend on hearsay and my birth certificate. I was a disappointment for my Mother who after having three boys, John, Beverley, and Oliver, had hoped for a daughter.

My Father was a family doctor and delivered me with the help of Mrs Warby, the acting midwife.

In due course I was christened at the parish church of St. Johns, Goose Green, East Dulwich.

Mother had so ardently hoped her fourth child would be a girl that she had tried by prayers to ensure her wish would be granted. She even had a wax doll which was beautifully dressed and which she nursed each day during her pregnancy, but alas to no avail. This disappointment for my Mother I look upon as my first undeserved "black mark." Others were to follow in due course in this story of my life.

There were others well deserved, which in my wisdom, I, have decided to omit. Earliest memory is almost impossible to differentiate from hearsay.

My first definite memory is when the family bought an Irish terrier puppy. This was such an exciting event that I can still see the frantic friendly greetings "Rob" had for everyone. He was the family pet. He lived for 16 years and died during the First World War.

At the end of the 19th century, I can recall a general sense of an impending unknown destiny. Of course I was conscious only of a sense of uncertainty. I now realise this was due to the beliefs of two groups of people. One of the ardent Christians who believed that the advent of the 20th century would herald Christ's Second coming. The other group had prophesied the end of the world!

In May 1900 Mafeking was relieved, the country went wild with rejoicing, and "Mafeking" became a figure of speech for years. This event is fixed in my mind because of the fireworks, illuminations and parties.

My next clear memory is of the death of Queen Victoria. I find it difficult to convey the countrywide heartache and sensation bordering on despair which created a sense of personal loss for each individual.

Our home had all the blinds drawn and everyone was silent and in mourning. Tearful eyes met one everywhere.

This proved to be far more the end of an era than the coming of the 20th century. "Life was never the same after the old Queen died."

However hope revived and energies recovered with the coming coronation of the new sovereign, King Edward VII.

All this optimism ceased abruptly and was followed by intense anxiety when he was taken seriously ill with appendicitis. The coronation had to be postponed. He was operated on and made a good recovery.

The nation rejoiced with thankfulness.

Amid countrywide rejoicing King Edward was crowned in Westminster Abbey with his beautiful consort, Queen Alexandra.

She was beloved by all for her kindness and consideration for everyone.

The King's recovery from appendicitis was the first recorded case and "appendicitis" became the fashionable disease and the number of cases, (real or imaginary) spread world-wide!

****

The day of the coronation was marked by amazing decorations and at night all window ledges were illuminated with coloured glass containers with lighted wax night lights. There were Coronation mugs, postcards, and even children's toys, and what thrilled me were the Coronation kites. They were square but flown with the corners pointing vertically and horizontally. With their very long ribbon type tails of brilliant colours, these kites could be made to perform all kinds of manoeuvres and were flown by boys and older enthusiasts in parks and on heaths and Commons.

Later, although so young, I remember people whistling or singing the popular tunes and songs of the day, such as the costermongers driving their small carts, or pushing barrows laden with goods.

This period of my early childhood was a particularly happy one.

My first cousin, May Robinson, was staying in our home.

She was years older, and I remember her with especial affection. It was a sad day for me when she left our home to start to train as a nurse at The Middlesex Hospital. Months later I heard that she was coming back one evening.

That night I kept awake hoping she would peep into the night nursery. She crept in so quietly that I nearly missed calling to her. She had not expected me to be awake. Even now this memory of her remains such a happy one.

She lived with us for years and for my Mother she was the daughter for whom she had longed.

My short period of school commenced soon after she left. I became a pupil at Modena House Kindergarten School. At first the teaching was not only interesting but so enjoyable. Learning under the Mistress of the juvenile class was far in advance of that era. We children enjoyed our lessons and we looked forward to them and adored her. She approached today's standard of education, which was then far in the future. I was apparently good at arithmetic and was soon promoted to a class of a higher age group because I could do long division. This eventually led to disaster!

Before that happened I earned my second undeserved (in my opinion) black mark.

It was the time of the annual Oxford and Cambridge boat race. We all had boat race favourites, either Oxford or the Cambridge Blue. That year the popular favours were miniature cycles with tiny pulleys as wheels. The cyclists were made from twisted pipe-stem cleaners, coloured light, or dark blue.

They were ingenious toys and when balanced on a string stretched across the room at a slight incline (i.e. a down gradient), they would apparently 'cycle' furiously across the room.

One of the pupils was an older boy. He was what would be termed educationally "subnormal" today, and he was determined that only Oxford favours could be worn and so he seized all the Cambridge ones and destroyed them! I was angry at this but could not physically tackle him, as he was so much bigger, and several years my senior! How could I get not only my own back but for the others as well? So I let all the air out of his bicycle tyres and was caught in the act! (Mark 2). The school was a two storey building. The ground floor was a large schoolroom and housed three classes. There was also a small section where hot milk, sometimes burnt, was given us during a break. I did not realise the significance that there was only one door for entry or exit. On the first floor upstairs was the Headmistress's room. Outside her door was a brass bell with a black handle. Pupils who committed a serious misdemeanour were sent from their class to report upstairs to ring the bell and await the dreaded summons to enter for judgement. On the whole, penalties were not too distressing, but the offender felt such an outcast. I became so used to being picked on, that the fateful bell lost much of its awe. One day the rumour spread that the Headmistress had retired and had sold the school. This proved to be true, and for me happy days ended. During an arithmetic lesson, I was in the higher age group when the new Headmistress entered. She looked with alarm and asked our mistress what is the meaning of this? These children appear to consider learning as a game.

The new Headmistress then pointed at me and said "What is that young boy doing in this senior class?

Our teacher tried to explain that she endeavoured to make her class enjoy their lessons, and that I had showed an aptitude for arithmetic.

The headmistress's reaction was devastating.

I was sent to the lowest age group, after an altercation between the new Headmistress and our beloved teacher. She was dismissed forthwith for failing to make her pupils realise that learning was a preparation for work in adult life and not for enjoyment.

This was such a blow to my self-esteem that I lost all interest in lessons. Especially as I had to do large cross-stitching on squares of cloth and was made to copy pot-hooks and letters on squared paper. No more arithmetic with my seniors. However, there arose another source of trouble which became wide spread, and that was using swear words. Most of these were quite foreign to me but, as so many of the children were getting into trouble, I thought of a way which would satisfy all. I invented a word which would mean all swear words, but sounded innocent. I got all my fellow pupils together and told them to say "DISMAGEW", when they wanted to use swear words. This word could mean: "Any swear words; damn, blast etc", I enumerated as many as I could remember. Nobody would know they were swearing. Unfortunately I was overheard by the Headmistress!

She thought she had caught the culprit and pooh-poohed my attempt to explain. (Mark 3).

My next black mark ended my kindergarten school career and I admit it was perhaps understandable but inexcusable. One history lesson was about the Norman Conquest, and in particular 'The Battle of Hastings'.

Before starting at Kindergarten I had learnt a description of the battle by heart from my Father.

'Harold had posted his men on the brow of a hill, behind a strong palisade. William, finding that he could not break the English ranks, ordered his left wing to turn and flee. The English charged after them, but the Normans suddenly turned round and attacked their pursuers with such fury that they were either slain or scattered in all directions'.

I considered myself an authority with my prior knowledge! So I suggested to my fellow pupils that we re-enact the battle. I divided them into Normans and Saxons and let battle commence! Unfortunately the result was a near juvenile riot and I earned my (4th black mark) at Kindergarten which ended my school career.

My conscience up till then had in no way worried me as I felt my intentions had all been for the good but had been misunderstood. So after being sent up to ring the brass bell, once more in disgrace, I thought why should I?

I decided to give the powers-that-be a taste of their own medicine. So I went quietly downstairs and unobserved opened the outside door and decided to go home. At this point I noticed the key in the door, and closing the door I turned the key in the lock and in a fit of temper threw it away.

This proved to be my undoing, for no-one could get in or out! Parents could not collect their children nor pupils get out. In those days there was no telephone, and it was not until one of parents fetched a workman to pick the lock that all were freed. This foolish act so tarnished my fourth. black mark that there was no hope of a pardon for such a deed. I paid heavily for this act. My parents were requested to remove me from the school.

Before I continue, I must mention my brothers. Jack was about 15, Beverley had died before I was born, Oliver was 11, and had had an accident, leaving him with a depressed fracture of the skull and was slowly recovering; Charles was about three and still in the nursery. I was in my seventh year.

Mother was in a quandary, when she heard that a Governess, of good family was free and willing to undertake the education and training of my younger brother and myself. I do not know what she was told, or by whom, but I think she must have had a report from or an interview with the headmistress of the school, for my new Governess told me that I was '*Satan's spawn*', and she had to 'drive the Devil out of me'. I had no idea what she meant, and I do not wish to stress her method of trying to reform me. It consisted of a beating each morning for the wicked sins I contemplated doing during the day and again at night for sins which I had committed. I was asked to confess each morning and night. Since leaving Kindergarten I had been confined to the nursery, except during the summer months when Father insisted that all his boys should learn to swim at an early age.

Father took us three boys to the local swimming baths during the summer months before breakfast. This was the one great joy of that time for me. I was not asked how I was getting on with my Governess and felt far too crushed to say anything.

One Christmas I was invited to a party by the mother of one of my old Kindergarten school friends. This was such an unexpected treat for me, as Jim had been my special chum.

My Governess took me to Jim's house and there was a changing room for guests to leave their outdoor things before joining the others.

I was very excited, but she would not let me go down to the party until I "confessed."

A stalemate resulted for I had nothing to confess.

This lasted until Jim's mother appeared to ask why I had not come down to join Jim and the others. How I enjoyed that party!

****

I will not continue to describe my Governess further as she was obviously unbalanced mentally, though she was well educated charming, and religious. Indeed she appeared to be the perfect governess and so she was to my younger brother. This situation continued for some years.

The end came when one day she seized a metal stair-rod and beat me with it. One blow landed on the crest of my hip bone 'to drive the Devil out of me'. This sharp pain was too much and I rebelled. I seized the stair-rod and beat her with all my might about her waist. Her waist was protected by her stays but the effect of my action was astonishing, for she rushed out of the nursery to run screaming downstairs in a state of hysteria.

This ended her career as a governess, but she remained for a time as a housekeeper, which was not popular with the servants.

There was one episode when I was under her care which is in retrospect so amusing that I will describe it.

My governess told me one day that a very important person was calling and she hoped to see the children.

She was Miss Ridley, of the same family as Bishop Ridley, the Martyr. I was drilled exactly as to how to behave like a Guardsman! When Miss Ridley arrived, I received my orders: "Geoffrey, advance! Salute Miss Ridley!" At first all went well, but Miss Ridley turned me round and I became disorientated. The final order came. "Geoffrey, thank Miss Ridley and retire!" I was to take three steps backwards, turn round and withdraw to the nursery. I obeyed, taking three steps back and fell head-over-heels down a flight of eight stairs!

There was for my parents the difficulty of what to do about continuing my education, and that of my brother, Oliver, who was rapidly improving.

A most fortunate solution arose. My Father was treating a retired Oxford Don, a classical scholar. He came partly for treatment as an in-patient, and undertook our education.

I shall never forget his kindness and the understanding way in which he taught us. He made every lesson an adventure and learning was once more a pleasant task. Under his tutorship we both made rapid progress and in the space of a few years we were both fit to sit for the Senior College of Preceptors examination.

Although I was not 16 until the last day of thc examination, I was allowed to sit and we both passed.

This success was entirely due to our tutor. Analysing and parsing he made into a detective game with clues and suspects. They could be any of the parts of speech.

I particularly recall his advice about translating English into French. "Never translate directly, but read the English version, make sure that you know all about it. Then put it away and write it in French. Think in French whilst composing." This may convey how thorough and explicit his coaching was, and how fortunate my brother and I were.

During these two periods after my leaving the Kindergarten, exciting changes were taking place. First, horse traffic was the only means of public transport for short distances. The age of the railway steam locomotive for long distance travel was at its zenith.

I remember how my governess had saved my two pennies a week pocket money. When she had enough, she asked my parents if she could take us two children on an excursion to Brighton for the day. The cost for adults was two shillings and sixpence. There may have been a reduction for children.

Early one morning we started off from Rye Lane Station taking a packed lunch with us.

It is difficult to describe the excitement and thrill of this adventure for young children. The hissing of steam, the banging of carriage doors, then the guard waving his green flag and blowing his whistle. We were off!

I was looking forward to swimming in the sea, especially as I held a badge for long distance, half a mile in fact, awarded to me by the Swimming Club at the baths. My nickname there was "The Shrimp."

That was during my kindergarten days. However back to Brighton! My ambition to swim freely in the sea there was too dangerous because of the breakers and different depths. I was put in the charge of an instructor who fastened a rope round my waist. (Wisely, though not in my opinion at the time!)

There were numerous bathers, and children paddling on the shore in the ebb and flow of the breakers' edge.

The life-line fastened round my waist was too short to allow me to get beyond the breakers so as to swim freely.

My attempts to swim were hazardous as each breaker would dash me on to the pebbles. For a short time I was swimming at last in a comparatively tranquil area between waves when a high breaker suddenly flung me violently on to the pebbles. I felt a sharp pain in my right foot. There was a shout of alarm from the instructor, and he pulled me out leaving a red trail behind. I had cut the sole of my right foot on a broken bottle. The bleeding soon ceased and a make-do bandage applied.

Then we had our packed lunch, but alas the glamour of the of the excursion had gone. I heard no more of the incident but was this another black mark ?

Naturally I was dejected for I felt my accident had marred what should have been a happy day for my young brother and myself.

We returned by train to our home and yesterday's world. Yesterday's world to me meant coercive domination by my governess ever since leaving Kindergarten.

From our day nursery window the horse buses were a welcome sight, especially the eight o'clock in the morning City bus; not the usual pair of horses, but a four-in-hand.

****

On May Day, the city bus was an inspiring sight; not four horses but a six-in-hand. All six horses were specially groomed with plaited manes and wearing cockades; they seemed so proud. There was no need for the driver to use his May Day whip with its white bow.

The conductor stood on top with a coach horn, which he sounded merrily to make the heavens ring!

When our tutor came, the era of the motorcar was just beginning. Horses were often scared and became panic-stricken, they would be almost beyond control. After a little while they became accustomed to the new era.

The 20mph speed limit was soon abolished, but for some years a man with a red flag had to walk in front of a working steam-roller.

I was learning to read before Kindergarten days. One day returning from the Dulwich swimming baths with Father and my two older brothers, we saw a steam-roller working. There was the man with the red flag emblazoned with the legend "Beware of the Steam-Roller." I was keen to show off my reading. Here was my chance. I stepped out and read as loudly as I could "Bravery of the Steam-roller!"

When we returned home, during breakfast my brothers described my 'faux pas' amid roars of laughter. My mother turned towards me and said with her amused whimsical smile,

"Oh yes indeed a steam-roller is very brave."

This was my first and effective realisation of the truth of the saying 'Think well before you speak'.

Later, I recall some humorous but trivial events. One is of the cats-meat man. His arrival with his small cart to our side-door was at once noticed by our terrier Rob, who as soon as he heard the sharpening of knives, would dash out of the kitchen door, and leap over the garden wall!

Father had taken pity on an injured jay, and this bird became a loved pet. It was a natural mimic and would imitate the call and the sound of the knife sharpening by the cats-meat man. Rob's response would be immediate. He must have had a sense of humour, for to us children he seemed to enjoy the joke so long as we laughed with him, not at him. He sensed the difference! The cats-meat man always had some tit-bits for him.

All the tradesmen called with their vans in those days. It needed simply to put Carter Paterson' card (CP) or Pickford's in the window, when parcels, or baggage would be collected by the carrier as he passed the same day or next, for delivery to any part of the country.

The coal-man's round was weekly; 1/6d to 1/10d a cwt, and I was aghast at the huge 2 cwt sacks carried by the men for delivery.

Our house faced Peckham Rye and we had an excellent view of all that took place on the common.

There was a bandstand and on Sundays and bank-holidays, during the summer numerous concerts were given by various bands, and we all enjoyed listening as the musical programmes of both popular, and classical melodies could be heard through our open windows.

Once when I was on the Rye, I saw an Airship very low and about to land. I was scared that it might explode! So I took to my heels, but as there was no sound as it landed, I plucked up courage and walked back cautiously. To my astonishment I saw the crew get out of the airship and hand ropes to bystanders, whilst the huge cigar-shaped gas bag was deflated. It was packed up and taken to the Peckham Park Manager's house. A few days later a lorry arrived with a quantity of gas cylinders. The gas bag was reinflated, and when all was ready, the airship slowly arose, the mooring ropes freed, then it gained height, and with engines working at full speed, it flew away.

This was some years before the first World War.

Mother's great friend was Mrs. Harley-Barker. She was a famous entertainer, and her son was Granville-Barker the actor and playwright. Mrs. Barker and my Mother used to entertain each other for hours rehearsing until each was so overcome with the other's rendering of humorous, tragic or heroic pieces of plays or poetry, that they would be reduced to tears! Father was a very practical man and he did not approve.

Mrs. Barker was the first person to broadcast and she did so over the whole of the United States.

At that time of course there was no radio, so the way in which it was arranged was by using the telephone. Subscribers throughout the network could apply to be plugged in.

Mother had a very large extensive repertoire and entertained people both at home or in halls with a multitude of recitations. They were not only well known works but she composed her own as well. She held audiences spellbound and was much in demand for charity events. Sadly this was before recordings could be made for posterity.

Gas was used with the old fish-tale burners for street lighting and in the home. When the gas mantle was invented and followed with a switch near the door to light the gas, how very up to date everyone felt!

Prior to that, to avoid going to the trouble of lighting the gas or taking a lantern, the senses of touch and smell were available to identify objects, clothing by brands of tobacco or scents, or by texture. There was much fun in the gloaming after a party. During the Autumn and Winter especially, roads became muddy, and mixed with horse droppings. This created a nauseous semi-liquid sludge, which was a source of concern for women with their long skirts. This was one of the reasons why a man walked on the outside to protect his fair companion from splashes caused by passing traffic.

Each street crossing had its own crossing-sweeper armed with a birch broom. His services were much appreciated by pedestrians who would award him.

A tip of two pence at that time was generous. With numerous tips on a busy day, the earnings would be well worth while.

The local councils provided special wagons with watertight bodies having anti-splash rims. Two men with long handled shovels would scoop up the sludge from the gutters to tip it into the carts. If a wagon was almost brimming, woe betide a passer-by!

There were coal fires in every house and the railway steam engines poured smoke into the atmosphere day and night. This produced those nauseous fogs for which London and the industrial towns were at times blanketed. Fog density varied enormously. I remember once seeing myself plainly as far as my knees but my feet and the pavement or roadway were quite invisible. During the worst fogs men with flares guided traffic and lost walkers. Coughing was the only indication that other folk were about. How thankful were folk to be safely indoors! One afternoon, when the darkened sky was threatening such a fog and we were glad to be indoors, we heard the muffin-man's bell as he rang it and called "Muffins and Crumpets!"

He carried a large tray balanced on his head, and the tray was covered by a large cosy. How we enjoyed rushing out of the house, stopping him to buy oven fresh crumpets for tea!

The roar and din of mechanised traffic were in the future, so sounds of life and happiness were audible in the streets.

Errand boys, and passers-by whistling or singing snatches of the popular songs of the day, with the cries of peddlers, all combined to fill the streets mingling in harmony with the tattooing of horses' hoofs.

The London Fire Brigade with their fire engines equipped with steam-engine pumps are now a forgotten sight.

The Dulwich fire engine, followed by the escape-wagon, would come galloping down Barry Road to the Rye when an alarm was received, the wagons swaying and the crews clinging precariously to their positions. Once the fire engine swerved on to the pavement and demolished our front gate-post. Fortunately there were no casualties.

The Annual London Fire Brigade Service was held on the Rye. A fake building 80 to 90 ft. high would be erected, then the teams would compete one after the other. The fire engines would gallop up with the hoses spraying jets of water to the top of the building, then the escape-wagons would arrive. The ladders would almost magically reach up to the top of the building. Firemen with their shining brass helmets would swarm up to the rescue of 'trapped people' and carry them down, a never to be forgotten demonstration of skill, daring, and courage.

On such occasions, and on Bank-holidays, crowds would gather and there would be a general merry-making. One summer we had a young German student staying with us on holiday. When he saw a merry-making on the Rye, he would say "In Germany that would not be allowed. Zee military would come down."

This rather annoyed us boys as these jolly crowds on the Rye were typical of Londoners 'On-the Spree', with abandon dancing so full of the good nature of the happy costers.

So whenever our young German friend would do something of which we took exception, we would cry: "In Germany that would not be allowed. Zee military would come down."

Little did we dream that in a few years' time 'the military would come down' with the advent of the first World War.

My father was a General Practitioner. He had a widespread practice, and a large number of his patients were of the deprived and poorest. This kept his income at a meagre reward for his long and hard toil.

In 1911, Lloyd-George's insurance act came into force. The popular ditty of that time was:

"Oh! Mr. Lloyd, now we are all employed!
Upon this little isle that we were born in,
And everybody but tramps,
Have got to lick their stamps,
And stick them on their cards, on Saturday morning!"

****

My mother not only performed many household duties such as the shopping, but also helped Father, by doing the dispensing of the medicines at the surgery all the week, and at the week-end made out the bills for medical attention. This was in addition to all the social activities she undertook.

The response of patients was very limited. Many tried to settle by barter, this helped slightly, but the strain was severe. Father felt that the New Insurance Bill meant financial disaster for the family.

When the first quarter's cheque arrived from the National Medical Insurance, we all realised that this might mean disaster. All at the breakfast table waited with intense anxiety as father opened the fatal envelope.

He drew out a cheque, looked at it and went quite pale, indeed he almost fainted!

The cheque was for an amount far beyond his wildest hopes and it represented for the first time an adequate reward for his arduous toil.

The whole family rejoiced for and with him.

I was a terror at wearing out my clothes, and one day Father took me to an Outfitters and bought me a cheap suit as a bargain. It looked well and the next Sunday morning I accompanied the family to the bandstand for the morning's performance. I was dutifully listening (rather bored in fact), when I saw a loose thread which I pulled and pulled, and rather to my amazement it grew longer and longer. Suddenly I felt chilly and looking down, my new knicker-bockers were just two flaps front and back! There was a hurried retreat home to the almost despair of my mother.

She quickly rallied and decided that the best thing she could do was to make me a kilt. This she quickly did in blue serge. I felt a bit awkward in this, but Mother pointed out that all the brawny highlanders in Scotland wore kilts.

Monday morning was the next day for the swimming baths. Father and we three boys started early for swimming. Jack was a powerful swimmer and was a member of the Barry Water Polo Team. We had great games pretending we were leaping off a ship-wreck. "Abandon ship! Women and children first!" Then crashing into the swimming bath in a higgledy-piggledy manner as though we were scared out of our lives.

Of course there were no girls, they had their own sacrosanct days.

On this particular Monday I was wearing my kilt. Father and my two brothers had gone on ahead. I and two friends of mine left later. After a while we heard ribald calls: "Is it a girl or a boy?"

At first I took no notice, but the provocative and spiteful remarks continued. My friends and I still ignored the tirade, but this seeming disregard was too much for the biggest of the three provokers and he sloshed me across the face with his wet swimming costume.

This was too much for me as well, and I shouted "I'll show you whether I am a girl or a boy!" and I knocked him down. Then I belaboured him with my wet costume. A passer-by checked me, and mindful of the Queensberry rules said, "You should not hit a man when he is down."

My reply was, "What on earth do you think I got him down for?" He laughed and walked off. Then I found that my assailant had taken the opportunity to disappear as had the other four.

Later I asked my friends where had they got to and their joint reply was "We were waiting for our tempers to get up!"

Father did most of his visiting patients on foot or on his bicycle. Rob the terrier was his constant companion on foot and he accompanied him on his twice daily attendances at the branch surgery close to Rye Lane, Peckham. If the weather was too bad, Father went by bus, and Rob would mount to the top to sit at the rear until the bus reached Rye Lane Station, where they would both dismount and join up to reach the surgery.

Rob was now getting old and in a few more years the journey on his old legs became too wearisome for him. He did not give up, but instead of following Father, he waited at the bus stop until the bus came, when he climbed the stairs to his place and he got off at Rye Lane Station. He was so well known that if there were no passengers waiting, the driver would pull up for Rob! When the horse buses were replaced by motor ones they still were Rob's devoted admirers.

Alas! The coming of the motor bus ended the reign of the 8 a.m. May Day bus.

The National Steam Bus Company started at a garage at Nunhead and was a source of wonder to the young. It was exciting to watch the efforts of the drivers working hard to raise a high steam pressure before starting on official routes. On frosty mornings, clouds of steam poured from each steam bus. Naturally the two bus companies competed. With a good head of steam, the National buses could draw well ahead, but if there were no chances of a stop to raise pressure again, the petrol buses would begin to catch up and perhaps overtake, to the cheers of youthful passengers.

Soon there were numerous motor bus companies in London, each painted in its company colours. This created a kaleidoscope of constantly changing colour combinations. Then they were all amalgamated into the London General Omnibus Company (all red). There remained almost up to the beginning of World War Two a solitary horse-bus which plied from Waterloo Station over Waterloo Bridge to the Strand. The fare was a halfpenny one way, one penny return!

The London County Council had an excellent electric tramway system with three rails, the centre rail being split for a 'plough', to make contact with an underground electric cable. I remember so well that on each tram was inscribed: 'Aubrey Llwelyn Coventry Fell, Tramways Manager'. This name always impressed me, as it seemed to cover most of England and Wales. There were cheap workmen's fares in the early hours. From about 11 a.m. till 4 p.m. it was 'Twopence all the Way'; a great boon for housewives, school parties, and the old folk. The busy housewives could shop adventurously, schoolchildren were able to explore the surburban countryside, as could the old folk. They were Cinderella outings, for the clock had to be watched!.

My brother Jack was an enthusiast for fireworks. Father took all the family to the Crystal Palace for the fireworks show. This was always a wonderful experience with 'set pieces'. Some of these were enormous. They included portraits of the King and Queen, sea battles with the destruction of enemy ships, boxing matches, and other subjects.

These firework displays with their showers of different coloured stars and volleys of rockets inspired my brother Jack, who got a book entitled 'The Pyrotechnist's Treasury'. This text-book gave complete detailed instructions how to make fireworks. I must give my brother full marks for the way in which he followed the rules for safety which he did in every detail. It was this care which in retrospect saved us from a possible disaster. For months we brothers worked as a team, each with his own job, and by Guy Fawkes day we had sufficient knowledge to give a display which, if not as brilliant as that of the Crystal Palace, was a fair imitation. There were Catherine wheels, flights of several hundreds of rockets, Roman candles, coloured flares, and mortar shells for showers of coloured stars. The only mishap was with a mortar shell during the experimental stage. These shells were made of compressed newspaper and were timed to explode and ignite the load of coloured stars at the maximum height.

The mishap occurred when a trial empty shell was fired. The internal explosion occurred during the shell's descent. A neighbour, an artist, putting the finishing brush strokes to his masterpiece of Richmond Yorkshire, was so startled by the explosion that it caused him to jerk his brush across the painting!.

Fortunately he managed to repair the damage!

He not only graciously accepted our apologies, but eventually gave the picture to my brother Oliver, and it now hangs as a treasured possession in my nephew's house at Cobham, Surrey.

What a supreme example of the 'good neighbour'.

However the years were passing and I was seventeen on the second of September 1913.

****

Then came the passing of the old year on New Year's eve. What did the new year have in store for us? The omens were of WAR. Every one hoped such a disaster could and would be avoided. I heard the New Year of 1914 being ushered in with a cacophony of foghorns in penetrating blasts by all the steamships on the Thames from St. Katherine's dock to Greenwich and Tilbury. There were added the cheers and good wishes from neighbours and complete strangers, all mingling as members of one family, accompanied with vigorous shaking of hands and singing "Auld Lang's Ayne." Then the toasting "To Absent Friends" and finally, tired out by the excitement, we wearily sought our beds.

As this is an auto-biography, I feel that I should stress the major events of my childhood, as they may have had a strong influence on my future.

My earliest years were of blissful happiness and left a memory of security and love during subsequent years.

At Kindergarten, my self confidence was severely shaken, when I found that when I tried to explain my actions at school. I was accused of telling lies.

The reign of my Governess started, as I mentioned earlier, in her belief that it was her duty to rid me of evil. She had an obsession that I was '*Satan's spawn*'. Her future actions were directed to free me from his spell.

One result was that I had the most terrifying nightmares.

The intensity and vividness with which I remember them in my old age shows the devastating effect that they had.

The worst illustrates my governess' tale of how 'Satan would come to claim me as his own!'

I awoke one night to see the window being slowly opened, and Satan's evil face watching me. He opened the window, and raised a large trident with which to impale me and carry me off. Then I would seem to wake up with relief that it was a dream, but as I watched, to my horror the window was again opened and this time Satan, waving his trident, leaped into the room. Such was my panic that I leapt out of bed and fled madly down four flights of stairs scattering my bedclothes in my despair, until leaping in mid air, I found myself embraced within my mother's arms. How she soothed and comforted me and drove all the horrors and terrors from my mind!

Alas I did not tell her the cause of such terrors, indeed I had no idea why they happened!

Later, the arrival of Walter Bazett, Esq. MA Oxon., our tutor, had a transfigurating effect on me. Gone were the threats of 'Satanic damnation'; he gradually restored my self-confidence. Soon after his arrival, and while my late governess was acting housekeeper, for some reason he left our morning session to go upstairs to change his shirt.

She, with a peremptory rap and instant opening of his bedroom door, was confronted by the spectacle of him pulling his shirt over his head. She had another attack of hysterical screaming as she rushed away downstairs. She would not confront him again for a fortnight and had all her meals alone. Soon after his arrival, our tutor took us, my brother Oliver and me, to the Tower of London. He was a tower of information, and, I shall never forget his descriptions of the sad history of so many of our finest statesman. Their sad advent through 'traitors' gate and beheading on Tower Hill. We saw the well known engraving by Sir Walter Raleigh on his cell window, made with his diamond ring: "Stone walls do not a prison make nor iron bars a cage." He took us to see the crown jewels and told us about their attempted theft.

I heard the tale of the jackdaws, that they would always remain whilst the Tower stood. I was watching the birds and for a time was alone, when a young couple approached. I suppose I must have been blocking their view, for he suddenly prodded me with his cane, and said in a la-di-da voice, "Out of the way, little boy."

I suddenly heard my voice saying, "Have you any idea to whom you are talking?"

He looked most embarrassed and his girl burst out laughing! Fortunately my tutor and brother appeared and all was well. W.B., (as we called him between ourselves), had an air of authority, which was perhaps just as well!

I was exceptionally short for my age at that time, and during the years of my teens under his compassionate tutelage, I shot up to a nearly normal height.

Our tutor stayed nearly up to the First World War. In 1913 Oliver and I sat for the Senior College of Preceptors and passed.

We could never have progressed so well as we did without his devotion.

Nevertheless, there are certain advantages associated with not attending school, and having private tuition at home. My eldest brother, John, went to school in the usual way, but my elder brother, Oliver, had had concussion of the brain following an accident. This left him with some difficulty of speech, and some temporary muscular weakness.

When our tutor took over, our ages were, John about nineteen, Oliver fifteen, and I was twelve, having left Kindergarten as already described. Our youngest was Charles, aged eight. So our tutor undertook the education of us three younger boys. He was an Oxford Don, W.B. Bazett, Esq., M.A. Under his benign rule we had much more free time, and we made the most of it! Father had got bicycles for us all, and he delighted to go for a ride with the family.

Dulwich Park, with its internal circular road, was just over a mile away, and after cycling there and back we were ready for Sunday lunch. This was but one of our family trips.

Unfortunately when the bicycles first arrived, the smallest was too big for Charles. So we had to devise a way of making it more his size. We had a reasonably equipped workshop, and could manage such jobs as cutting steel, tubing, and brazing joints. We made the bicycle smaller by cutting two inches off each tube of the triangular main frame, then joining them together again with steel collars, making the joints secure by brazing. When finished, Charles could ride his bicycle with ease and safety. We were foolhardy in the way we recklessly rode our bicycles within our garden.

We even cycled along the tops of the walls, each of which was one brick (lengthways) wide. We tried to play a crude game of polo and in addition raced madly around the garden.

The result, apart from some minor bruises to ourselves, was damage to the bicycles. Front wheels were the main casualties. I fail to have any idea as to how many buckled front wheels we managed to repair by fitting new spokes and somehow reducing the distortions in rims. Father finally decreed that if we were not more careful, he would not replace any more damaged parts. It must have been when I was about 15 and Charles about 11, that the time we feared eventually arrived. Charles skidded on his bicycle, and his front wheel was hopelessly buckled. As regards cycling, Charles was now immobilised.

It was then that the idea of the 'Trandem' was conceived. This was to remove the ruined front wheel from Charles's bike, fit the front forks of his machine over the axle of the back wheel of mine. This was not as easy to do as it appeared.

The front forks had to be separated wider than usual, care being taken not to overstrain. Then the holes were too small to fit over the back spindle of my bike. They had to be enlarged, and finally the front forks were bolted successfully over the back axle of my machine. Charles's front brake had to be discarded.

So far so good, our three wheeled 'Trandem' was complete.

We soon found that to ride it was not simple, and we had to relearn how to balance it, how to steer, and especially for the rear rider to accommodate his power pedalling.

We soon became adept, but we appeared erratic when pedalling, as the gear ratios differed for the front and the back riders. The front gear ratio was comparatively high, whilst the rear was lower. Thus, when in action, the front rider pedalled fairly slowly, while the one behind had to pedal faster. On long trips, when on a slight decline, pedalling for the rear rider became too rapid and he would have to free wheel. When going uphill, if the rear rider was too vigorous, his half of the machine would try to overtake the front with the predictable result of catastrophe!

We became 'show offs', and used to demonstrate how we could come to a halt, and remain stationary with the machine partly folded on itself, while we remained upright on our saddles.

Filled with enthusiasm, I fitted on the front handlebars a bell similar to those on the horse fire-engines. These brass bells had a strap attached to the clapper, which the bell-ringer would energetically operate to clear a way for the engine.

We decided to try its effect one Saturday afternoon when Rye Lane, Peckham, would be crammed with shoppers. As we entered this busy shopping street, I rang the bell as fast as I could. I was unprepared for the result! A way suddenly opened up for us, as people panicked, and parted, mothers snatching their children, whilst men pulled each other out of danger, as our tandem cycled cheekily past.

We deserved to be berated at least for causing such a commotion, but not so! There was a large Cockney element in the crowd, and our so sudden and alarming arrival was treated as a huge joke. I doubt if today such a hilarious reaction would be possible. Our tandem had become an object of curiosity. We refused to let the unwary try to ride it, because of its peculiar totally unexpected habits. It was far too precious to risk in the hands of novices!

Naturally we had become so used to its caprices, that to onlookers it must have appeared as simple as ordinary cycling. One day two of our friends decided to try it when we were not about. They grabbed the tandem, mounted both saddles and attempted to ride off. They were completely at a loss as to how to control the machine, because of the difference from riding a two wheeled vehicle. They crashed badly, completely wrecking our precious tandem, by buckling the front wheel and bending the front forks. The damage was irreparable and thus ended the 'Transom's short but amazing life cycle'.

****

We had hoped to make another, but Oliver and I were sitting for our pre-medical course examinations. I was 16 during the examination. Our tutor had retired. Charles went to Dulwich College, and our happy-go-lucky free times were at an end. However, we had had numerous successful excursions on the trandem. We had cycled 'Tandemised' to Hayes and Keston and other picnic places, and these memories will be with us always.

Our tutor stayed nearly up to the First World War. In 1913, Oliver and I sat for the Senior College of Preceptors Examination. I was only permitted to sit because my 16th birthday was on the last day of the examination. To the credit of our tutor, we both passed. To our regret, owing to ill health, he had to give up and retire.

Early in 1914, my brother Oliver and I started a preliminary course at King's College, Strand, before starting the university first year Medical Course in the Michaelmas term.

The threat of war increased, so we joined the University O.T.C. "Square bashing" or infantry drill started with parades on the square of Somerset House next door to the college. We for the first time heard remarks far from complimentary about our physique, mental status and future.

Easter found us in camp on Salisbury Plain. This we found exhilarating and exciting, especially as the international situation grew more and more menacing.

The summer of 1914 was lovely and all the seaside resorts were crammed.

Yet at the back of everyone's mind was the fear of war, it was always there.

During the summer vacation, the O.T.C. was in camp again training hard.

On August 4th we heard with mixed feelings that war with Germany had been declared. The overwhelming feeling was one of intense patriotism and the fear that it would be all over before Christmas so that we cadets had little chance of fighting for King and Country. I read an article by a financial expert who predicted that the cost of modern war was so vast that all wealth would be exhausted and the protagonists would be bankrupted into collapse within a few weeks!

Patriotic fervour was huge and widespread throughout the country. Camp was cancelled and we returned home to await news as to what would be our next personal orders.

My eldest brother, Jack, was qualified and House Physician at King's College Hospital, where he met his future wife, Hetty Woolvern, a trained King's College Hospital nurse. My brother, Oliver, was soon commissioned as second Lieutenant. Royal Fusiliers, and was posted to his unit at Shoreham. I remained in a state of limbo awaiting my 18th birthday in September. I was unaware of how unprepared I was for army life, in fact I was an 'ingenue', having missed the rough and tumble of school life.

In the meantime, I was free to make the most of my leisure before being called up. Buses and trams allowed free travel for soldiers in uniform. Accordingly, the short period I had of 'leave' I made the most of by exploring London and its environs. My younger brother, Charles, was continuing his education at Dulwich College.

Early in November I had an imposing communication from the War Office informing me that I had been given a commission as second Lieutenant, 14th Middlesex regiment, and that I should report forthwith to the Regiment's barracks at Gravesend.

****

Having reached the magical age of 18, I was full of ambition to achieve almost heroic feats for 'King and Country'!

On reporting to the barracks at Gravesend, I found that the battalion was in the process of formation. I was the first subaltern to be appointed. This gave me seniority over all those commissioned later than I had been.

Unfortunately, I was too naive to take advantage of this almost unbelievable fortunate start.

Seven days leave to have my uniform made was allowed and I returned home. An army tailor in Chancery Lane fitted me out, and before reporting back, I had my portrait in uniform plus swagger cane taken!

When I returned I found an amazing change.

Many more recruits for Kitchener's army had arrived, and the battalion was rapidly building up to full strength. They were volunteers mainly, but also a few transfers from other battalions of other ranks, whose loss would not be regretted. One of my first duties was the early morning run, we started at full strength, but such was my enthusiasm, that when we returned to barracks there were two sergeants, three lance/corporals and only about a dozen privates left! The C.O. was not impressed, nor the Adjutant! They pointed out that if I continued in this way there would soon be no battalion left!

About this time, there was a rumour that enemy spies were everywhere, and people were asked to report any suspicious characters. This was unfortunate for anyone with a name of possible German sounding origin.

The result was that many Jews, who were undoubtedly loyal citizens, were unfairly suspected to be spies. Probably these doubts would soon have settled down, but drinking, gossiping and scandals soon excited mobs, which gathered outside shops with Germanic sounding names, and were followed by outbreaks of looting.

In Gravesend, the Superintendent of the Police feared that the situation might get out of hand and he telephoned the barracks to ask for support of the army to prevent the rioting spreading.

It happened to be my night on duty, and I was told to take my company down to the town centre to help the police.

I had arrived only a few days before, and I was ignorant as to how the army should tackle a civilian disturbance.

My detachment, 'all present and correct', duly paraded, and marched out of barracks, down Parrock Street towards the Clocktower Square. When we were about 100 yards from the square, I wondered what the most effective action would be to take. So I halted the column and ordered "Fix bayonets," then: "At the double surround Clocktower!" "Halt!"

The result was not exactly as I had expected, but the effect was instantaneous. The police had already got control but when my mobile column appeared on the scene with fixed bayonets, the square emptied as if by magic, except for the police.

The police superintendent thanked me for the contingent's quick arrival. With unfixed bayonets my heroic column returned to barracks.

I had done a terrible thing. The army is not allowed to march with fixed bayonets. It was contrary to King's regulations.

Ignorance is bliss, so it is said, but that did not prevent me being told in no uncertain terms not to repeat the offence. Officers began to arrive from Territorial battalions and from the City of London Rifles. Most were far more experienced and older than I. Full Lieutenants were naturally senior to me. One was a barrister about 35, and he was inclined to develop a severe stutter when agitated or anxious, which increased his stuttering until he became incoherent.

This weakness became known to the recruits and they played him up. When he was drilling a squad on the parade ground, and he became agitated, he was 'fair game'.

One day he had a bunch of unruly recruits who were inclined to treat drilling as a joke.

****

At first all went reasonably well, but soon the laxity of the squad became a source of anxiety, and his stuttering began. This became worse and worse as the squad deliberately began to make errors. When he ordered "Right turn", some would, others did a left turn. He had the squad marching towards a high wall but efforts to shout "About turn!" became almost inaudible, and when disaster was imminent, he managed to cry: "Stop you damn fools! ... STOP!"

The squad managed to halt in time and then started to laugh like a lot of schoolboys. Not for long, for the door of the orderly room opened, and the second in command of the battalion appeared. He was a retired regular officer on the reserve and very much 'ON DUTY'.

The startled change in that squad into one of sheer fright seemed to me to be miraculous. Gone was all the slackness, and after they had been sufficiently disciplined, the squad was handed over to the battalion Sergeant-Major! No squad ever played up like that again.

I was given command of C. Company, and felt I was doing 'my bit' as the saying was. Yet I certainly felt embarrassed when I was leading C. Company along the High Street one day, and a motherly type of woman called out "Just look at that young boy! It's a shame!"

C. Company at once responded by singing: "You're my baby! Oh what a wonderful child!" My face became scarlet as we marched.

One of the senior captains was asked by the C.O. to lecture the subalterns on how to behave, so as to maintain the dignity and honour of the King's commission.

The meeting was duly held, and all we junior officers attended. Finally he warned us not to speak to any girls in the street. In my innocence I asked why. I had spoken to one the other day and she was most helpful! He looked quite shocked and said,

"I am sorry to hear that. Do not do so again."

I replied I had wanted to post a letter and I had asked her where the post office was. This remark of mine caused roars of laughter from the subalterns, and I think our mentor was convinced that I was taking the Micky out of him.

A few days later I was orderly officer, and accompanied by the orderly sergeant, visited the men at breakfast to ask if there were any complaints.

One of the men got up and said,

"Yes Sir! These eggs are not fit for human consumption. They are all bad, look at the nasty green rings inside them."

At once cries of disgust arose from others. Soon they started banging their spoons, and creating quite an uproar.

They had spotted they had a 'ninny' as orderly officer. I should have asked for an egg, eaten it, and said it was good. Such a commotion followed until the Adjutant arrived and settled the matter by eating one of the eggs himself. The battalion soon moved to Snodland, Halling and Darenth areas to prepare a trench system for the outer defence of London. This was a wooded, hilly and charming countryside. The digging of trenches with precautions against possible accidents was more than interesting. A definite distance had to be kept between men digging trenches, so that the swing of a pickaxe or other tool could not possibly injure the next in line. Careful inspection of trench walls was routine. I was returning one evening after visiting my section. This area was reached by a narrow bridle track with high banks and sharp bends. There was no room for one vehicle to pass another except where there were passing bays.

I was near the junction of the lane with the major road when I saw one of our men lying unconscious across the track in a dangerous position. It was now quite dark, and I tried to move him to one side. With the dimmed lighting of wartime vehicles, even if I managed to do so, his position would still be perilous.

His breathing was stertorious, his breath smelt of drink, I tried to get him on his feet but he was too far gone.

A company vehicle was due at any moment, so using 'the fireman's lift' I got him over my left shoulder and carried him to the guard room in the major road a few yards ahead. I handed my burden over to the sentry saying to the Sergeant "I found this, look after him, please," and returned to the Mess. Again I had erred, I should have put him on a charge. Apparently I had somehow not behaved in a manner befitting that of an officer holding His Majesty's Commission, but no alternative was suggested.

I was feeling uncertain as to how to live up to the standard of an officer and gentleman, when I was asked to report to the C.O, as I had broken King's Regulations. Whatever had I done now? I asked myself, and when I duly reported before the C.O., I found that all my brother officers were there. Everyone looked ominous.

The C.O. said,

"Robinson, you have broken King's Regulations," and he handed me the orderly room copy opened and said,

"Read the paragraph number indicated."

I read: "Officers must not shave the upper lip."

Everyone in the room except myself burst into peals of laughter. I had a fine fair down of an embryo moustache which had yet to feel the touch of a razor.

Actually this was intended as a humorous joke. I quite failed to see it that way and felt self-conscious and humiliated.

Next morning very hopefully, I started daily shaving the upper lip!

It was now late in the year, and Christmas was only a week away, when I was given a week's embarkation leave before posting to France, as a replacement for a casualty.

Full of excitement at this news, I happily started off to spend an unexpected Christmas at home. My brother Charles and I had an enjoyable holiday, though neither of our two older brothers were at home. Mother and Father made a great fuss of us, and I left home; with their good wishes ringing in my ears. Two days before I left home, I had a sore throat and felt not at all well when I said goodbye. The train journey was slow and very cold. When I arrived at the Mess I felt feverish, giddy, and could hardly swallow. My draft was to leave in the morning. I rang up the battalion M.O. and asked if he would see me as an emergency.

This he did, but when I explained about the draft, and I feared my sore throat might stop me going. I said would he give me something to buck me up?

I noticed he was swinging a lead pencil between his fingers and then gave me a long lecture that it was a privilege for the country's young men to serve their King and Country. He appeared quite disbelieving.

"Cannot you at least take my temperature?" I asked.

Rather grudgingly he did so. When he looked at the thermometer he ejaculated "Good God." The next thing I knew I was in hospital and missed the draft.

Unfortunately a brother officer had to take my place and go without embarkation leave. Although I felt I was in no way to blame, I felt in a way responsible.

On the whole I managed quite well at Gravesend and was beginning to enjoy the army life, but soon the battalion was ordered to Colchester for further training.

My batman was a middle aged Irishman who was full of 'blarney'. The day of the move I was to report at 6 a.m., so I told him to call me in good time. Next day I was awakened by the Adjutant's orderly. I had missed roll-call and got a severe dressing down.

When I tackled my batman about not calling me in time his excuse was:

"Sure it was meself who came well in time to call you, but when I sees you lying there just like my own son so peaceful and quiet, I tried hard, but I just couldn't force meself to wake you, to do so would have broken my heart"!

I never saw him again, and I am sure that he was a scamp. He also should have sent on my regimental trunk which contained my spare uniform, extra clothing and my sword.

I had no idea what to do following this loss, which seemed to amuse all the mess. It was a complete financial disaster and crippled me for months. Looking back, I realise that I was considered a 'Sissy'. Especially as I was a non-smoker, and a teetotaller, not at that time out of conviction but because I just did not like smoking nor alcoholic drinks.

I felt too insecure to make a fuss. What advice I did seek was no real help.

Soon I was due for leave once again. I left barracks for the station and I was cheerfully looking forward to home. I showed my leave pass and hurried to get a seat as the train was just starting.

Can you imagine my alarm when I heard loud shouting:

"Is Lieutenant Robinson there?"

The train was starting to move, so I put my head out to ask what was the matter.

"You are under arrest!" shouted a Sergeant of the Military Police. This was more than I was prepared to stomach. I said

"I am on leave and shall be back in six days!"

As the train gathered speed, I expected trouble when I got to Liverpool Street, but all was well, and I got home to a warm welcome. I kept quiet about the incident.

When I returned from leave, I had to see the C.O., who told me that some of my cheques had been returned marked R.D., in other words they had 'bounced'. I was dumbfounded as I had been particularly careful to avoid such a catastrophe. Cox's, the army bankers, were unable at first to understand how the situation could have occurred, as my cheque book counterfoils did not agree with cheques debited to my account.

However there was a Lieutenant Robinson in the 15th battalion and our two signatures were almost identical, if signed in haste. They were Geoffrey W. Robinson, Middx. Rgt. and George W. Robinson, Middx. Rgt. Both were debited to my account. Cox's apologised and I thought that was the end of this error.

I changed my signature permanently to G.Waring Robinson.

This unfortunate incident disturbed me and I wondered what other mischance might befall. I was not left long in doubt. I had hired a motorbike whilst mine was being repaired. I had thought that to get to know the Colchester area would be a help when manoeuvres began.

On a Saturday afternoon, I collected the hired machine and started off. I had not gone far when I saw that the High Street along which I was travelling was crowded with shoppers. I attempted to slow down to a walking pace. To my alarm the throttle wire snapped and instead of slowing the bike began to pick up speed. The brakes failed to stop the machine and I found myself beginning to hurtle towards the crowd. I put my hand down and turned off the petrol but realised it would take too long before the bike stopped. My only hope was to snatch the high tension cable off the sparking plug. My hand shook with the electric shocks and I started to wobble. With a violent jerk I managed to break the connection. The motorbike rapidly lost speed but not soon enough for me to control the erratic wobbling. Frantically I tried to gain control which I did as the machine came to a halt leaving me off balance, when I found myself steadied in the arms of a woman shopper. I was quite enfolded in her motherly arms as she controlled not only me but the machine as well.

She was so sympathetic and understanding, and dismissed my attempts to make abject apologies. Her hands had saved me from a nasty fall, and I realised how fortunate I had been. My relief was short, for a Constable appeared with notebook!

My rescuer at once came to my aid. With an intensity that surprised me she said: "Officer, I saw it all! This young officer tried his utmost to avoid an accident. He could not have done more."

The Constable thanked her, but pointed out that he had his duty to do.

With a kindly expression he started to question me:

"Are you the owner of this machine, Sir?"

I replied,

"Not exactly."

At once the kindly look faded and was replaced by a suspicious gleam in his eyes.

"Your name, unit, and address, Sir, and your driving licence, please."

I said,

"My licence is in the barracks, and I hired the motorbike whilst mine is being repaired."

"Who is the owner, and which garage?"

I was not sure.

"The garage is up the hill and is the one which sells Pratt's petrol," I answered.

By now the notebook had copious notes and the Constable appeared less suspicious and said: "I shall have to report this to the authorities." He then bade me "Good-day", and left.

Fortunately the machine had an ordinary bicycle chain and pedals, so I was able, wearily and slowly, to pedal back to the garage. The owner-manager had left, but the lad who was selling petrol told me my machine was ready. So I was able to ride back wondering what would be the result of this new misadventure. Next morning the Brigadier sent for me. As soon as I reported he said,

"Are you not the officer whose cheques were bounced?"

The Adjutant said,

"That has been satisfactorily explained, Sir."

The brigadier had a list of the motor offences I had committed the day before, and was more than annoyed that the Civil Authority had complained.

He told me not go on my motorbike into the town in future but to confine its use within army precincts and outside the town. Then I was dismissed with a wave of the hand. I noticed an amused smile on the Adjutant's face as I saluted and left. After the morning's parade and mid-day meal I had a little time on my hands.

There was a seductive appeal about the motorbike.

Yesterday I had been too 'on edge' to appreciate any extra performance. The parade ground was deserted, so here was an ideal occasion! I started the engine and vaulted on to the saddle thrilled with the purring of the twin cylinder Douglas horizontally opposed engine. Definitely improved, I made one circuit and decided to make another. I was nearing headquarters and starting to make a left turn, when of all people the brigadier stepped out of his office.

I was not too near him but decided to make a tighter turn. The front wheel skidded on loose gravel and down the bike and I went. I stopped in a sitting position at the brigadier's feet. I was in dread of almost unbearable condemnation; instead he helped me to my feet so considerately, grabbed my hand, which I had grazed, and said,

"Go to the M.I. room and have that injury treated straight away." His attitude was almost paternal! My opinion of the brigadier went up by leaps and bounds. This episode went round the mess and I enjoyed the banter.

Although I felt, after this experience, more self confident, I was anxious to avoid more set-backs. In fact I was far from being self-reliant!

The brigade was ordered to the rifle range for practice and to test ability. I hoped that I would do reasonably well. When my turn came, I was so distracted by everyone watching, that I developed a severe intention tremor, with the result that my first shot was so off target that it landed on the next in line. I was taken off and had to shoot on my own.

So when my solo effort came, everyone gathered round to watch. Though my efforts were an improvement in spite of my anxiety, they still were erratic, and provided amusement to the onlookers. My score was pitiable. Then we had 'sharp-shooting'. The target would appear for a second and then disappear. I had to shoot on my own of course. When the target popped up there was no time to dally and as soon as I saw and aimed, I fired. Such a roar of laughter greeted my shot! I had scored a bull. The laughter ceased as the next was an inner, for when sharp-shooting was over, I headed the list for sharp-shooting in Brigade Orders.

Everyone congratulated me, and my tremor disappeared. Next came the Brigade cross running race. I came in 23rd, which out of about 2,000+, was reasonable.

Next came map reading and sketching. All junior officers were told to make a sketch from the top of a hill and mark suitable positions for artillery to shell an imaginary enemy. Mine was chosen as the best and used for demonstration.

At last I felt that I had shown that I was of full value as a member of the mess.

Soon after the rifle practice, rumour ran round the brigade that we should soon be embarking for France, and that an extensive field exercise was to be held almost at once.

This was correct, and we were all hoping to demonstrate how efficient as a fighting unit the brigade was.

It was now May, and the countryside was a riot of Spring blossoms with early bright greenery.

Beforehand, we were all lectured on procedure, to obey orders at once without question but at the same time be ready to act on one's own initiative if the situation clearly so demanded. This tail-bit impressed me, as I had been reading an account of the Peninsular War and the value of seeing an error in the enemy's disposition by an alert junior officer.

The Guards were to be the enemy and their positions extended by planting scarlet flags.

All went according to plan. I was acting Captain when I suddenly saw a gap in the enemy lines. To advance and cut the enemy line in two appeared to be an amazing opportunity, and mindful of "acting on my own initiative", I ordered my company to advance under the shelter of a defile to occupy and seize such an important site.

I noticed some of my junior officers (but senior in age) laughing but I thought nothing of that.

Then I saw a staff officer on a white charger galloping towards me "Who the Hell is in charge here?" he shouted in fury.

When I said I was, his language was too damning for me to attempt to repeat.

My action had so upset the battle plan, that the exercise was abandoned.

I was told to report back to barracks, and to remain in my quarters pending a decision at H.Q.

An inquiry was held, and came to the conclusion that either I had been too careless to bother, or that my action was deliberate to 'avoid the column'. Someone pointed out that I had 'dodged the column before' after taking embarkation leave, and a brother officer had to take my place and forfeit his leave. Eventually the choice lay between my facing a court-martial or being dismissed from my unit and sent to the O.T.C. at Shoreham for further training.

I am sure that it was my C.O. who saved me from the disgrace of being court-martialled.

The unit left for France and the Battle of the Somme; whilst I feeling distraught reported to the O.T.C. at Shoreham.

My hopes and ambition had been shattered and I felt that there must have been some unexplained reason for my humiliation. I consulted King's Regulations and found that if an officer felt aggrieved, he could apply in confidence to the Military Secretary at the War Office for advice.

So I wrote and eventually saw a Staff Major at Whitehall.

To my surprise he was sympathetic and said he fully understood how I felt. Then he pointed out the nation was fighting a war of survival and time was not available to spare for everyone.

Then he suggested that, as from my records I was a registered medical student, I should apply for permission to resume my medical course and leave the combative forces.

I thanked him for his advice and returned to Shoreham, where thinking over the interview I felt two aspects were important. First I had had a fair hearing. Secondly if I applied to resume my medical course, would this not be interpreted as a third effort to 'Dodge the Column'?

This second option was intolerable so I returned to Shoreham hoping I could do better.

At first all went well, and I expected to be posted to an active unit in the near future.

The O.T.C. was stationed on the South Downs and the hut allotted to my section was at the bottom of a slope. When it rained for several days we had to wade through water as the hut was flooded. A most unpleasant experience when getting into bed.

During the Autumn my health suffered from recurrent attacks of tonsillitis and I became debilitated.

A special army exercise had been planned in which we were to compete against a regular force. Naturally we were keen to show how efficient we were. This was in the afternoon of a damp day, and after parading at the map reference on the top of a hill, we waited and waited but no opponents appeared. It started to rain and a cold wind made us all wet through. Finally we were told the exercise was cancelled but we were to await orders.

Soon transport arrived and we were offered the choice of taking the evening off with transport to Shoreham or we could opt to attend a lecture at H.Q. I and a few others opted for the lecture. We were told transport would soon be here. There was more waiting and I began to feel giddy and faint. The prolonged standing about was grim and finally I collapsed and fainted. When I recovered we were already back in our quarters and I went to bed.

Next morning I felt much better and heard that the C.O. wished to see me. He said "I have heard from the police at Shoreham that last night you created a disturbance by being drunk, kissing the Sergeant-Major and behaving uproariously!"

I noticed an amused twinkle in his eyes and of course I had opted for the lecture, so I had a perfect alibi.

It was not a Robinson this time but a Lieutenant Robertson who acted so hilariously. This escapade made him very popular among the subalterns and he escaped with a mild censure and advised to cease kissing his Sergeant-Major.

Life at Shoreham proceeded normally for some weeks and I will not mention minor happenings during that time.

My hopes of doing well began to fade and I wrote to my Cousin May who had married a Surgeon R.N. to ask if there was a chance of my transferring to the Royal Naval Air Service to train as an air pilot.

To my great relief her husband, Rear Admiral R.N.M.S. Robert Stewart, arranged for me to be accepted for training as an air-pilot if my medical examination was satisfactory.

In high spirits, I attended at Milbank Royal Naval Hospital for this opportunity at last to vindicate myself.

At first all went well and I was congratulating myself, when I only had the eyesight examination left. Again I did well until it came to colour vision.

I failed the Eldridge-Green lantern test and the colour bead test. I could not believe this and attributed the result to colour ignorance. In response to my anxious plea I was given another chance to attend for a further colour vision in a month. This result confirmed the first, and in the midst of my almost darkest gloom of depression, there came a sudden clear revelation of certainty: 'This caused my failure on that field-day'. I had 'four' colour vision, instead of the normal five'. I was practically green-blind, and I could not detect the difference between the yellow-red of scarlet and the yellow-green of spring foliage.

The warning flags in that area to me were invisible.

Looking back now, it seems extraordinary that no one, including myself, thought of this possible explanation.

Freed from the possibility of 'Dodging the Column' concept, I could now, with a clear conscience, resume my medical studies. Indeed, I received every sympathy from H.Q. at Shoreham and was given six months 'sick leave'.

Fortunately, this coincided with the start of the Academic Year at King's College, Strand, and I was able to take the first medical MB, BS. examination within three months and could then start the second year's course in 'Anatomy and Physiology'.

This was the period of the Zeppelin raids over England; they did more damage than is realised nowadays. This threat was soon countered however by the Royal Army Flying Corps, aided by searchlights and anti-aircraft batteries.

One evening in October 1916 such a raid on London was in progress with numerous searchlights and air raid warnings. I went out on to the Rye, and there high in the sky was a Zeppelin, brilliantly lit as it was trapped in focus by the converging searchlights. Suddenly I saw a biplane, which seemed so tiny compared with the huge airship, attack the Zeppelin. Then a small flame appeared on top of the airship. Rapidly, it spread. Soon the Zeppelin was ablaze from one end to the other. All the intricate tracery of the metal framework was clearly visible. The Zeppelin came down at Cuffley.

I jumped on my cycle to pedal madly north over the Thames. At last I reached the spot where it had come down. There it lay, a huge twisted still smouldering heap.

I kept a piece of one of the radiators; curiously, this was lost when our home was bombed in World War Two.

During these raids, anti-aircraft fire was so intense, that falling shrapnel came whistling down and was a danger in itself.

Never shall I forget the ghastly yet amazing brilliance of that doomed Zeppelin, when the zenith seemed ablaze and all London was bathed in the reflected glow of the lurid death throes of the airship.

At Cuffley a stone memorial at the site records the event.

It was at King's College Strand that I met my great friend Gerald Rudolf. Through his friendship I met his family, they lived near the hospital. I was received by them as one of their own. His father,

Prebendary Rudolf, founded the Church of England's Waifs and Strays Society, later re-named 'The Children's Society'. Gerald's elder sister, Dorothy, undertook the almost impossible task of teaching me to sing in tune. She did have a modicum of success as there were not so many pained questioning glances directed at me if I dared to join in a hymn or in a student sing-song! She was Secretary to the 'Waifs and Strays Society' and later to King's College Hospital fund raising department in the days of the Voluntary Hospitals.

During the early stages of the war everyone was asked to help combat any possibility of gross food shortage.

Gerald told me one day that he had read an article advising people near lakes or ponds to stock them with elvers 'young eels'. They would grow during the summer and provide nourishment. There was a small lake, (or large pond), in a private piece of land which could be rented reasonably for this purpose to help the war effort. It was near North Dulwich Station, so, enthusiastically, we rented it. Then we found that the only place to get elvers was in Germany. However we had the use of the land. I heard of a derelict punt at Richmond, whilst it was not fit to use on the Thames, which would be good enough for our lake. It was a long arduous trip pushing a barrow with such a lengthy, heavy load, but it was worth it.

The punt was a success and was appreciated by all.

The lake and its surrounding parkland became a favourite haunt of students and friends from the hospital.

One day I was swimming in the lake, when a passer-by on the path outside stopped and peering over the hedge, called out to me: "A donkey was buried where you are swimming"!

This fact rather took me aback but I replied

"Can you swim?"

He answered "No."

"Come on in then, you would be company for him!"

He made no further comment and walked off.

However the swimming no longer appealed, whether or no his remark was true. Certainly I decided not to do any underwater exploring!

Fortunately for me, the start of my eight months' sick-leave coincided approximately with the start of the academic year. The first year dealt with biology, organic chemistry, and electro-magnetism. I already had some knowledge of these subjects, so, working hard, I was able to sit for the first year's M.B., B.S. examination after three months. Thus Gerald Rudolf and I started the second year's course together.

I cannot let the first year's course go without mentioning one incident, which occurred during a practical zoology class under Professor Dendy. He placed in front of me a glass bottle saying "Draw that."

There was the perfectly preserved cartilaginous skeleton of a dogfish. It was in excellent condition on a black background. I decided to copy it as perfectly as I could. So I decided to have the white skeleton shown in relief on the black background within the bottle.

I was keen to get the effect I thought suitable by careful shading. I was admiring the result when Prof. Dendy returned. He took one look at my drawing and almost bellowed with wrath "Damned art!" and departed leaving me somewhat deflated. Of course he wanted an anatomical diagram.

We as a class were (unlike the 'Old Queen') indeed amused.

At this time there were numerous students from India, Egypt and other countries, also third year students from the forces who had been given leave to continue their medical studies. Casualties among unit M.Os. had been unbelievable. A unit's M.O. had been given a staff like a patrol leader in the Boy Scouts, with a Red Cross pennant at the top. He, with this non-combatant emblem, was to succour the wounded in no-man's land. The staff, with its Red-Cross pennant, was no protection for snipers would fire at the slightest movement. So all senior medical students in the forces were told to resume their medical courses.

The number of women students rapidly increased. I was struck by the energy they put into taking copious notes. I confess that I envied them this aptitude. They were following the full academic course, whilst we had to qualify as soon as possible for the forces. (Some excuse!)

I took the second medical at the end of my leave, so could start clinical studies with Gerald at King's College Hospital.

In fine weather we always walked to the various hospitals for special diseases.

Distances were between about five miles and twelve miles.

There were visits to schools for the deaf, the blind, and for the mentally ill or retarded.

This was soon after the 'Lunatic Asylums' had been renamed 'Mental Hospitals'. As regards public health, we visited water reservoirs, drainage systems, and sewage treatment filter beds. At that time, sewage treatment was so efficient, that visitors were invited to drink a crystal-clear pure water from the final standing water hydrant. Since then, all these centres have become overloaded due, to population increase and the use of agricultural fertilisers.

The City of London Mental Hospital at Stone, near Dartford, Kent, was our longest walk.

These expeditions were in addition to ward rounds, lectures, and note taking of in-patients at King's.

In fine weather, Gerald and I met for an early morning 'run' before starting for the hospital. Whenever possible, if our clinical studies took us elsewhere, we walked. This meant 12 miles to the City of London Mental Hospital, Stone, Dartford, to hear lectures by Professor Steen. He was an excellent teacher and his patients received every care. Sometimes all the students would join in these pleasant walks.

The South Eastern Fever Hospital at New Cross was much nearer, being about 4 miles.

Whilst at the college in the Strand, there were so few students that we were unable to play team games, when we started at the hospital, our numbers were sufficient.

I enjoyed being a member of a team. Being so few before, we had to make do with 'runs' and paper chases 'Hares and Hounds'. One occasion I remember particularly. Gerald knew the Chiselhurst area well and arranged for one to take place there. He and I were the hares and set off laying a 'trail' of bits of paper. Sad to say, we upset a local authority road sweeper when we laid our paper trail on his recently swept pavement. His remarks were vibrant with scorn to put it mildly.

Looking back at our finances at that time makes the result of inflation very obvious. My daily allowance for the day was two shillings, (10p today). On this I travelled from Dulwich to the Strand and back, had lunch and still had some change in my pocket. However, in spite of inflation, I am sure with the amazing modern methods of mass production most things are cheaper today, with the exception of railway travel.

Which recalls to me a vague memory of a journey by the 'tupenny tube'. I must have been very young but I remember that foul hissing foetid, sulphurous fumes seemed to be all pervading.

Life at the start of the 1914 war, and especially before conscription, was difficult for young men 'in civvies'. One day I had taken a seat in a bus for the hospital, when I felt a touch on my shoulder, I turned round and there was a marvellous girl looking at me. I thought 'The Fairy Princess!' I know that it may be difficult to believe that I was so ignorant, but when she handed me a white feather, I had no idea of its significance.

"Thank you indeed, how very kind of you" I said as I put the feather with pride in my hatband.

I noticed that she seemed puzzled at my response and pleasure. An elderly man rose and was about to say something to me, when the bus stopped and he had to get off.

You can imagine the roar of laughter when I got to the hospital and told about my meeting with the 'Fairy Princess' and learnt its true meaning!.

So I joined the R.N.A.S.B.A.R. in full Royal Naval Auxiliary Sick Berth Attendant Reserve and wore a navy blue armlet embroidered with a red anchor.

I had no further trouble in that way but I never saw the "Fairy Princess" again.

Looking back to those training days, I realise what amazing advances have been made in medicine and surgery.

In surgery, the recent war had revolutionised the treatment of fractures, burns, lung injuries (due to gas warfare), and the repair of severe facial injuries.

One example shows how indebted we all are to the progress in preventative medicine.

When we attended the Acute Infective Diseases (Fever) Hospital at New Cross, we saw children suffering from scarlet fever, whooping cough, and the most fatal of diseases, diphtheria. The children suffering from diphtheria were in two wards. In the first ward the children were not allowed to make the slightest muscular effort that could be avoided in their cots or beds.

The nursing staff did everything possible to prevent their small patients exerting themselves in any way.

A high degree of nursing skill was needed and was an early form of today's intensive care.

The reason for this was the dread of heart failure due to paralysis. The healthy 'lub dub' of the normal heart beat would change to a clocklike rhythm 'tic-tock'. If this dreaded change occurred, the child was moved to another ward, where there was no restriction on movement in bed. Toys were allowed so the child could enjoy a little happiness before the heart suddenly stopped beating.

At that time there was nothing which could be done to avoid a fatality. When I hear objections to innoculations, I recall to mind those bereaved parents. At this period antibiotics had not been discovered, and deaths from such diseases as tuberculosis, rheumatic fever, and bacterial infections, were frequent. The first lifesaving drug was sulphonamide, which saved so many from death in cases of acute pneumonia, and some other infections. Then with the arrival of penicillin the whole aspect of medicine changed. The full benefit was not felt until World War Two was over.

Whilst in the third year of our clinical education, all of us students witnessed the first intravenous injection of a drug. The patient's arm was shaved and carefully prepared forty eight hours beforehand. The students and nurses had to wear masks and gowns. We all held our breaths as the physician inserted the intravenous needle, and then injected the drug.

This great care today may seem extraordinary, especially as so many bloodlettings had been done in the past.

The explanation of the precautions was quite simple. It was felt that the injection of a foreign body into the blood stream might cause massive blood clotting and death. Earlier attempts at blood transfusions had in most cases ended fatally. During the last years of my clinical training, I had frequent attacks of tonsillitis, and I determined to have my tonsils out as soon as I qualified.

Gerald and I qualified in 1920, and I entered the E.N.T. ward at King's for tonsillectomy. The operation took place next day, and, apart from some slight bleeding, I made a quick recovery. The E.N.T. houseman was Dr. Lawrence, who later became the eminent authority on diabetes. He had the misfortune to have a speck of bone lodge in his eye while operating. The resulting small corneal ulcer would not heal and he had to go sick. It turned out he was a diabetic, which was the reason for the ulcer not healing. When the cause was found he was treated accordingly and recovered in due course.

Meanwhile there was no houseman to look after the E.N.T. patients. On the third day after my operation, I got up and acted as his temporary locum-tenens. As he could not resume his duties, I was offered this senior house job and accepted it. This six months in the house led to my deciding to specialise in 'Oto-Rhino-laryngology', at least part-time, and I applied for the post of Assistant to the E.N.T. out-patient department.

I was accepted and attended for two afternoon sessions a week. This was of course a voluntary unpaid job but it carried with it some prestige.

My eldest brother, Jack, when the war ended returned to civilian life. He had served thoughout the war in the navy as Lieutenant Surgeon on a cruiser and was on station off the coast of East Africa. He was present at the surrender of German East Africa by the German forces.

After the war he returned home to join my father in the general practice on The Rye.

My elder brother was posted to Belfast near the end of the war. He was able to resume his medical training at the medical school there and passed his first and second years examinations.

When peace was declared he returned home and started his clinical final years at King's College Hospital, qualifying in the early twenties.

My younger brother Charles had caught pulmonary tuberculosis from a patient when acting as dispenser at the branch surgery. He became seriously ill and had years of treatment in hospital, both medical and surgical. His convalescence was long and tedious.

Yet he took out a correspondence course and studied for a degree in Higher Education. After qualification, he was appointed Lecturer at a Polytechnic College. He was much missed when he had to retire after many years of teaching. My Father now had three sons who were qualified and able to help and expand the practice.

In addition Jack had his Diploma in Anaesthetics. Oliver, a keen photographer, took his Diploma in Radiology.

So we three brothers formed a team and were able to do surgical operations of a minor category either at a patient's home or in the surgery.

One day I saw an advertisement in the British Medical Journal for a Junior Medical Officer at the City of London Mental hospital.

Professor Steen was still the Superintendent.

I applied for the post with the approval of my Father and brothers. After an interview with Professor Steen, the Hospital Management Committee appointed me to the post of Junior Medical Assistant Officer.

The medical Staff consisted of Professor Steen, a Senior Assistant Medical Officer in charge of the female side, and the Junior Medical Officer looked after the male side.

The Hospital had extensive grounds, with playing fields and a farm which supplied dairy products, fresh vegetables and fruit. There were cricket, tennis, hockey, and football teams in which those patients who were well enough took part.

Among the male patients were some famous characters; a renowned composer of music, an artist who had been an illustrator for Punch, and many children's books. Also a doctor who regularly admitted himself when he felt an attack of his mental disorder was pending. The work was at first astonishing and it took some weeks before I felt confident. It was an eye-opener to find out how much care was taken of the patients, they were interviewed on the daily ward round. Every week a report of each patient's condition was written up in the case book.

Also each patient was regularly seen by Professor Steen.

Under the Mental Health Act each patient had to appear before a Committee from the Ministry for review, (I believe quarterly), so that no patient who was mentally capable was retained against his or her will.

Professor Steen persuaded the Committee of Management to purchase a house outside the hospital grounds where patients who were making good progress towards normality, could manage to look after themselves with a minimum of supervision. Over 80% of them eventually were able to resume life with their families. When the Senior Medical Officer was away, the Junior took over his duties. In due time I was called on to do his daily round. This was my first visit on duty to the female side.

The Senior Nursing Sister or Charge Nurse awaited my arrival and conducted me into a large day room.

To my surprise, Sister left me standing in the centre of the room amid a most peculiar feeling of tensed expectancy; for all around the wall of the day-room, patients were seated, most of them gazing at me.

Anyone in these circumstances would feel a bit self-conscious and I was certainly no exception.

Suddenly one of the patients jumped up and took several steps towards me. She pointed an accusing finger at me and shouted at the top of her voice,

"That is the man who ruined my sister!"

At first I was uncertain how to react to this accusation but I soon realised that I was not the first to be blamed for whatever disaster had befallen her sister!

Charge sister reappeared at my side, and amid much amusement, explained that this episode was a regular happening which would lose much of its entertainment value if newcomers were warned beforehand.

Most patients were too introspective to have common interests but this one amusing incident was enjoyed by many of them. This introspection prevented patients from forming friendships and from planning any joint action.

One patient's delusion was that she was Queen Elizabeth I and she was very regal in her behaviour.

Curiously on my first visit she was being very difficult, and refused to have her regular bath. She stormed at the nurse

"We will not have a bath!" resisting all efforts to make her change her mind. Her refusal was physical and she was adamant in her regal displeasure.

Charge nurse appeared and summoned reinforcements.

Her Majesty was in no way dismayed but drew herself up and commanded,

"We would have a bath, see to it forthwith!"

So her royal prerogative was not infringed.

One day I failed to recognise one of the male patients, he appeared so normal both in his demeanour and speech.

"Are you the doctor in charge of the ward?" he asked.

"Yes," I replied.

He then told me that he was being illegally detained against his will and that he was instructing his solicitor to take out writs against Professor Steen and me. All his other remarks seemed to me so sensible that I asked Professor Steen about him. The Superintendent advised me to see him tomorrow morning.

The next morning I had to ask the Charge nurse where he was. When he was brought for examination, I would hardly have known him. Yesterday's spruce and indignant personality was replaced by an almost incredible vacancy of intelligence.

If a patient became threatening it was a rule that he should be restrained by several nurses acting in concert. This avoided a patient injuring himself or others.

One patient would eat his clothing so he had to wear a shirt made of tough ticking. There was one man who nearly choked himself by attempting to swallow a ticking shirt. He had to be put in a warmed padded room so as to protect himself from himself, clad as he was born.

Tranquillisers had not been discovered but their eventual use was a great step forward and subsequently led to many patients being able to return home to be cared for by relatives.

One night in summer the weather was oppressive, and distant thunder echoed ominously. My bed was a double one with large brass knobs at the foot. I went to sleep quickly but was suddenly awakened by a terrific flash of lightning. I found I could not breathe and I was conscious of the receding diminishing rolls of thunder. My heart was racing, I could not inhale, and two huge iridescent globes of violet-blue light apparently replaced the brass knobs.

Eventually my breathing restarted with rapid shallow inhalations. This was a great relief and soon I felt much better. What impressed me was that I had not heard the original clap of thunder.

When I had recovered enough I got up and looked out of the window. Lightning had struck the roof gutter and 'earthed' down the drain pipe beside the bedroom window. The pipe was split, torn from the wall and lay partly incinerated across the path outside.

The hospital farm was famous for its pigs: 'Kent Middle Whites'. Every day a quart jug of full cream milk was placed on my table. That, and the traditional English breakfast of fresh milk with bacon and eggs, caused me to put on weight from my normal ten stone to twelve. I played hockey for the hospital, also cricket and tennis. I missed the regular morning runs, so I decided to cut down on this tempting diet.

Breakfast and tea were meals in my rooms, for lunch and dinner I was invited on a permanent basis to Matron's flat to join her, the Assistant Matron and her husband who was the Senior Assistant

Medical Officer. Conversation was largely about local activities and of course 'shop'.

Then it would take on an atmosphere of gossip about personal acquaintances.

"I wonder what Eddie is getting up to ?"

"Whatever it is, George will put a stop to it unless he takes care!"

"It will all depend on Mary's approval."

I was at a loss, until one day I realised the conversation was about the Royal Family. I felt rather 'out of it' but one day the maid tapped at the door and said to Matron,

"Lady Robbins is on the telephone and wishes to speak to Dr. Robinson."

This boosted my ego!

Lady Robbins was the widow of the late Sir Edmund Robbins who founded the Press Association. The family were near neighbours and had been my Father's patients, and family friends for years.

My appointment at the City of London Mental Hospital carried a good salary and for the first time in my life I was independent. I had reasonable time off and could attend the out-patients department at King's College Hospital two afternoons a week.

This appointment was to prove most fortunate for me as it was there I met my future wife. This delightful meeting was yet to be, and will be described later.

It is difficult to describe what an amazing change socially it was for me to mix with young people of both sexes, who were so uninhibited in jovial friendship.

During the Voluntary Hospital period there was a different atmosphere.

We all worked for the benefit of the patients, none of whom were left unseen however late we had to stay. There was no clock watching, but there were rare breaks when we could rest for a few minutes and enjoy a cup of coffee or tea with a bun or an Eccles cake, this last was a special favourite. These lulls were filled with a sense of puckish euphoria and happy camaraderie.

The W.V.S. (Women's Voluntary Service) had a refreshment stall which was very popular with patients of all ages.

The Great War had ended in 1918, and the Nation's relief after the terrible losses each day, food rationing, and now the welcoming home of young children from evacuation, led to a widespread national feeling of optimism which was the background of the 'Gay Twenties'.

Between the two world wars during the twenties and earlier thirties all forms of art and entertainment with plays, and poetry flourished. Jazz musicians with famous bands played for us all on radio, in dance halls, and in cinemas. Truly this was the period of the 'Gay Twenties'. It was the era of the 'Bright Young Things' and the then modern youth had one foot in an "Austin Seven", and the other in a "Gypsy Moth"!

Finally in the thirties came the appalling world financial crisis, with, as already mentioned, the rise of Hitler the dire threat of Nazi Germany.

****

I thoroughly enjoyed my afternoon sessions at King's but there was one particular occasion which remains ever fresh in my memory.

I had occasion to seek some details about a patient in the E.N.T. ward.

The telephone was answered by the staff nurse on duty. She had such a delightful voice that I hoped I would have the opportunity to meet the owner of such a charming voice. This ambition was unexpectedly realised, for 'the power that be' decided to appoint her as staff nurse to the E.N.T. out-patient department.

I had been entranced by her voice but when I met her I was forever enchanted.

I had to find a way to talk to her quietly without incurring the displeasure of Sister.

Any hint of a budding romance between a nurse and a houseman or clinical assistant, such as myself, was severely frowned on, and might lead to a nurse having to give up her training.

So one afternoon I left a bottle of chromic acid crystals on my table 'forgetfully'. Then next afternoon when there were no out-patients, (and I knew she was on duty), I returned to collect the precious bottle, so 'accidentally' left on my table. (At this point please refer to my wife's autobiography). Our friendship rapidly developed into a lasting relationship. Rennie took me to meet her relatives at Sidcup. They were so kind and I looked forward to further visits, especially as Rennie's Aunt Beatrice whispered in her ear "I like him"!

Of course I was not supposed to hear, but with joy and pride I did.

We had many outings together when off duty time permitted, and after several anxious proposals, she agreed to marry me, and we announced our engagement to our families, but we had to keep it secret from King's !

I invited her to see the City of London Mental Hospital and introduced her to Matron, the Assistant Matron, and her husband the Senior Medical Assistant.

Sadly, about this time Professor Steen had a heart attack and was in another hospital for observation and treatment. Cardiology was still in its infancy. Indeed I do not think it was a recognised speciality.

Later he returned to duty but was never quite the same robust person.

Tragically, Professor Steen had another heart attack from which he never recovered sufficiently to resume his duties and, to the sorrow of all the staff, he died.

Meanwhile, I had noticed that possibly patients who heard voices or claimed that they were being persecuted by "wireless", were in some cases suffering from diseases of the ears and might be misinterpreting tinnitus or noises in the ear.

I decided to do some research on this subject.

If true, then treatment of the underlying ear condition might show that the hallucinations were in fact delusions and in some cases help patients towards recovery.

In addition to the patients already under my care, I saw patients from Maudsley hospital at King's ENT out-patients, also I visited Claybury Mental Hospital where my friend, Gerald Rudolf was now a Senior Assistant Medical Officer, later the Superintendent.

He was one of the first to do research 'shock' therapy for certain mental disorders. After one of my visits he asked a patient,

"Did the Ear specialist help you?"

She replied,

"Oh yes I can now hear my dead sister much more clearly"!

Today, with the 'tranquilliser' drugs and psychoanalysis, many patients have reason to be thankful for the long and detailed research done by pharmaceutical firms and also to psychiatrists. The hospital had a huge entertainment ball with a stage and proscenium, in fact an excellent small theatre. Some of the patients were able to avail themselves of the chance to forget their peculiarities for a time by either taking part in productions or enjoying them. A play which went down well was 'Browne with an E'. Rennie was able to see one of the performances.

This inspired me to try my hand at writing a playlet with Rennie as the star.

I had done some amateur conjuring and decided to use it in the playlet.

The theme was that of an Ancient Egyptian love story between a Hebrew slave and Pharaoh's daughter, 'The Princess Loti'.

I managed to hire the gown worn by Evelyn Laye as Cleopatra.

This exquisite costume fitted Rennie perfectly and here in all her beauty was my 'Fairy Princess', let alone Pharaoh's daughter.

The plot was about an Egyptologist returning from archaeological excavations in Egypt, who brought back the sarcophagus and mummy of the Princess Loti, together with her empty treasure chest. In the play they are prominently on view with a statue of the Egyptian god Ammon Ra and two chairs. The Egyptologist is describing to a friend the story of how the love affair was discovered and both the lovers were put to death. There is an inscription written within the chest which the Egyptologist has to get into the chest to decipher. He reads that there is a curse on anyone who treats the princess's memory or belongings with irreverence.

There is a crash as the treasure chest lid suddenly falls and the locking clasp closes.

The friend hurries to raise the lid, when he suddenly exclaims, "The mummy has disappeared!"

There is a gentle tapping from within the chest. The friend unlocks the clasp and the treasure chest lid gently lifts and the Princess Loti appears.

She recognises the friend as the reincarnation of her lover. The friend is bewildered and emotionally confused with dormant memories which are so poignant and inexplicable. He attempts to greet her, but the time gap between them prevents them from meeting physically and the friend collapses.

The Princess Loti is distraught and kneels at the statue of Ammon Ra and prays "Forgive us both, the Past and the Present."

The Princess bows her head, then occurs a 'thunder clap', a brilliant flash, and the stage setting is as before.

The Princess has disappeared, the mummy is back in the sarcophagus and the two men are sitting in their chairs. The friend says,

"I have had a wonderful experience, was it a dream? I saw the Princess Loti."

The Egyptologist rises and taking centre stage says,

"We have met the dead!"

Curtain.

The playlet as a play was a success, but two patients in the audience had hysterical attacks and were taken back to their wards. One member of the cast was a patient and he played the part of the friend of the Egyptologist. He was very good and he did it very well. Shortly after the performance, his recovery was complete and he returned to his home.

Soon after this performance, I was told that the Management Committee would like to see me at their next meeting. So I duly attended to find that the Chairman, Sir George Truscot, was unable to be there. Sadly, Professor Steen had died and I lacked his backing at the meeting. The Acting Chairman raised the subject of my engagement and pointed out that there was no accommodation for a married junior assistant. I replied that I was aware of that but that there was no early prospect of our marrying. He then asked if it was true, as he had heard, that on my free afternoons I attended the E.N.T. out-patient department of King's College Hospital? If so, why? This question seemed to me to be unreasonable.

I replied, "I understood that I could use my free time as I pleased."

He said, "That is not the point, but it appears to me that you are taking advantage of this hospital to study another branch of medicine."

By this time I was indignant and retorted "If I spent my afternoons in hunting, fishing, or shooting, or some disreputable amusement such as gambling or drinking, that would cause no adverse comment."

This rather unwise remark upset the Chairman. It was at this point that the late Professor Steen would have spoken on my behalf. My senior colleague was silent.

The Acting Chairman said "It appears that you are not really interested in Mental Diseases and that it would be better for you to leave, especially as there is no prospect of the hospital providing married accommodation."

So ended my appointment at the City of London Mental Hospital. Obviously I was not at my best when answering loaded oral questions from the Committee. I also felt that my expression had changed to that of childhood's embarrassment, when my governess used to say, "Geoffrey confess!"

I heard later that my successor was too fond of the bottle and when he left, accommodation was provided for a married medical officer if required.

So I returned to General Practice with my Father and my two brothers.

****

The Great World War had ended in 1918, and the nation's relief after the terrible losses each day, food rationing, and at last the welcoming home of the children who had been evacuated, led to a widespread national feeling of optimism which was the background of the "Gay Twenties."

Optimism after victory was universal among the Allies. The Treaty of Versailles bore heavily on the defeated. Emphasis on reparations rendered the Weimar Republic powerless to control the demon of inflation.

The German financial world collapsed and their people became desperate. The United States and Great Britain between them lent Germany more than £1,500 millions to help repair the wreckage left after the war. This left many still hopelessly unemployed and formed a breeding ground for Hitler to exploit, by organising the unemployed and German Youth in his campaign, "Strength through Joy."

He formed troops of young men to revitalise agriculture. In addition, he arranged holiday tours on cruise liners to proclaim his campaign. This was an appeal which found an echo and sympathy among many people in this country and others. The sudden vilifying of the Jews, with its ghastly sequels, revealed Hitler's evil megalomania.

Offers for asylum for the oppressed were made from many countries. My wife and I offered a temporary home for a refugee, and a Jewess managed to get an exit visa on the strength of our offer. She stayed with us for some years and helped in various ways. She was an excellent bookkeeper.

Of her family she was the only one to survive. Her brother and sister were famous operatic singers and both perished in Hitler's dreadful concentration camps.

Back to the earlier "twenties." The enthusiastic revival of civil life expressed itself by means of numerous pageants of local and historical interest. These were held in villages and towns which produced local talent of surprising excellence and inventiveness. Usually they were historical, recalling the local history from pre-roman Britain, Roman, Anglo-Saxon and the Norman conquest up to near modern times.

In Bexley, Kent, there was the story of (Joan), "The Fair Maid of Kent", who lived at Hall Place. She was the Countess of Kent, and as her popular name implied, of surpassing beauty. She was the widow of a cousin of Edward III, and eventually married the Prince of Wales, the "Black Prince."

Their only child was Richard II, the boy king, who is renowned for his courage during the Peasants' Revolt, when Wat Tyler was wounded by Mayor Walworth, and killed by an equerry of the King. This alarming crisis was met by the young king, who rode forward alone with the cry: "I will be your leader! You shall have all you seek! Only follow me to the fields outside!"

The event was commemorated by the naming of the site Walworth Road after the Mayor.

This was a central event in Bexley's pageant, which ended with an amazing portrayal of Hitler and his storm troopers by a patient of mine, who was a Jew.

The salary I had had from the Mental Hospital enabled me to employ a secretary for Father's practice, thus freeing my Mother from dispensing and much of the practice accounting. At first we managed well for we did minor surgery, and four to five E.N.T. operations for fees which suited individual patients. Also I had consultative and operative sessions for local authorities.

The Children's Hospital for sick children at Sydenham advertised for an Assistant Ear, Nose and Throat Surgeon, for which I successfully applied. This honorary position was important because it enlarged the scope of operating. So Rennie and I felt that we could fix the date for our wedding.

One memorable day Rennie and I, while visiting her relatives at Sidcup, went for a long country walk to North Cray, where we explored a country lane. We came across a vacant cottage to let.

Enthusiastically, and perhaps heedlessly, we signed a lease for three years. There was a large garden with fruit trees and a rose pergola.

With almost childish glee we burnt paper in the sitting room fireplace and rushed out to see smoke coming out of the chimney of our future home!

One day I saw an advertisement in the Daily Telegraph for a Government Sale by Auction of Surplus Surgical and Medical Materials, following the end of World War I, at Shepherds Bush. I decided to go to the sale.

The quantity of material was enormous, condition was faultless and the successful bids were ridiculously low.

I bought two portable operating tables and a quantity of instruments for merely token sums and returned home astonished at my good fortune.

We fixed the date for the wedding to take place shortly after Rennie finished her training, in December 1925. I was afraid that if she had accepted the offer of the hospital to go to the nursing home in Monte Carlo run by King's College Hospital followed by missionary work abroad, I might lose her. Rennie's uncle, the Reverend Benjamin Payne, was very fond of his favourite niece, and both families were delighted when he not only offered to officiate, but invited us to spend our honeymoon at his Vicarage in Dovercourt.

December arrived, and Rennie shared top with her friend Miss Seth-Smith of that year's nurses training class.

Although far from affluent, we went to Harrods for our furniture. I will not go into details but we purchased some excellent things which we still have.

Then came the bedroom furniture, and I foolishly chose two single beds. My parents had single beds and I thought this was quite usual. I noticed the salesman seemed a bit taken aback, Rennie was far too shy to suggest the obvious alternative. There was the usual hustle and excitement as our wedding day, the 19th, drew nearer and nearer. Apart from other things, I purchased a smart pair of new shoes.

All my wedding apparel I took to North Cray the night before.

****

It is an ill wind that blows no one any good, as the saying goes, alas the converse may also be true.

Suddenly, a few weeks before our wedding 'The Hospital Savings' scheme started and had the effect of seriously reducing my income whilst I had to work harder in the voluntary service. The General Practice relieved me of the secretary's salary, which eased the situation to some extent.

Gerald Rudolf was to be best man, my future father-in-law was to give Rennie away, and her sister Eva was to be bridesmaid. Waking on the morning of the big occasion I was beset with anxieties, and particularly mindful of my Father's advice: "Always remember and never forget that your wedding day is the most important day in the whole of your life."

Looking at my reflection whilst shaving that morning I marvelled at my good fortune; I still couldn't quite believe it. The marriage service was to be at twelve noon. I was on my own in our cottage, The White House, and after a hasty breakfast I washed up and tidied our future home best as I could. I had carefully laid out my 'Moss Bros Outfit' and started to dress.

What on earth had I done with the ring? This was near panic until I calmed myself and thought back. Of course. It was in my attaché case, and thank goodness, there it was. I had finished dressing but for my new shoes which would complete my outfit. It was about ten o'clock. The shoes were still in the car wrapped in paper. I picked up the parcel and found to my horror there was only the right shoe!

Frantic now, for time was passing, memories of nursery days flooded back: "Geoffrey comport yourself." So I did, and systematically I searched the car. No shoe to be found. Then I considered what other footwear I had available at our cottage. There were four pairs: the shoes I had driven down in, (which were brown and there was no time to blacken them, even if I had the blacking), bedroom slippers, (which were black but too incongruous, even with spats), a pair of Wellingtons, (quite impossible), and lastly an old pair of gardening black shoes. I routed them out and found them very soiled from working in the garden. I remembered that, soon after buying them, I had damaged the toecap of one so badly that I took the shoe to a cobbler to see if he could help. This was during World War 1, a time of make do and mend. He patched the toecap with fine stitches and it was the left shoe.

With spats it would have to do. I cleaned the shoe as well as I could, but it had a peculiar shade of decay. I lit a candle and collected some of its soot and with a true army mixture of spit and elbow grease I produced a passable polish. True, there was still the patch with its radiating fine stitches! It would have to do nonetheless and might pass muster with the spat carefully arranged.

By now, it was zero time, if I hoped to reach the church before my bride's arrival.

Of course all eyes were anxious to see what the bride would be wearing, so for some time I escaped scrutiny.

Worn out by the morning's anxieties, I was near despair.

The bride was late, due to the chauffeur's insistence that it was her privilege.

I was so worried that I was barely aware of Gerald's presence, that of my mother and father, Rennie's grandfather, or of the gathering of families and friends.

Gerald asked me for the ring and I must have handed it over, but I was scarcely conscious of doing so.

Suddenly, to my almost unbelievable relief, the church door opened and there was my bride in all her purity and loveliness, escorted by her father and sister bridesmaid.

I saw only Rennie and failed at that moment to appreciate her lovely bridal dress or to marvel at the beautiful bouquet of white lilac in December, yet to my subconscious mind they enhanced perfection.

After the homily the marriage service continued with the usual responses, but when Rennie was about to answer "Yes," she caught sight of the now shining patch on my left shoe and it took the most superb control on her part not to giggle.

As newly-weds we retired to the vestry to sign the register and on our return, Rennie's Aunt Lois spotted my shoe and remarked "Something old and something new."

Outside we gathered for congratulations, photographs and well wishing.

The reception was at Rennie's Uncle Frank Walker's and Aunt Beatrice's home at Sidcup. How we appreciated their kindness, generosity, and hospitality.

For me the relief from that day's earlier troubles was bliss.

We all enjoyed chatting with one another and laughing. No two families could have come from such different backgrounds. The Paynes were all associated with the Christian religion. Rennie's grandfather was a doctor of Divinity, Dr. Thomas Payne. He was the author of numerous theological works and was well known on both sides of the Atlantic. Her father was headmaster of a Protestant Mission School in Dublin, and her Uncle Benjamin, who married us, was a Church of England vicar. Our host at the reception was editor of the Methodist magazine "Foreign Field."

The Robinsons were rather a boisterous family and at the reception were bent on enjoying the good fare.

Grandfather Payne suddenly arose and said, "Let us have a word of prayer."

The Robinsons were so involved in talk, that some failed to hear the summons at first. There was some spluttering as they hastily gulped down their tea and tried to kneel gracefully. This in no way disturbed Rennie's grandfather, whose praying soon impressed everyone, with its message of family Christian love and its petition that our marriage would in due time be blessed and future generations would recall this day with thoughts of family love embracing all the generations.

Time was passing and I had to think of the drive to Dovercourt which was about a hundred miles. So far the weather had been fine for December, but rain was imminent, and as we gathered about the car, I started to raise the hood and fix it, when the shoe shot into air and fell with a plop onto the pavement!

Then the heavens opened and in a deluge we drove off.

I was of course driving so Rennie's Uncle Ben did not feel too 'de trop' during the journey to Dovercourt. Rennie and I were looking forward to our arrival there and the greeting from Ruth, our hostess, Ben's wife.

The modern road traffic conditions were in the far distant future. He who reached the crossroads first had the right of way! So there would often arise the question 'Who was first?' I remember helping to extract one of the first Austin 7's, with its two occupants from a haystack, at a crossroad. They were none the worse, nor was the car for the experience. Speeds were much less and few motorists could exceed an average of thirty five miles per hour on a long journey. Casualty figures however became terrible. Road deaths in one year totalled nearly 28,000 and led to the Road Traffic Act. However all went well on our honeymoon trip, and on our arrival at Dovercourt, Ruth's welcome, (in which Ben now joined) is one of our treasured memories.

Next morning, we went down to the shore of Dovercourt Bay, which in December had a charm of its own. There were long sandy beaches and the countryside adjoining was picturesque with its sand dunes and waving reeds, interspersed with dykes for drainage and a number of windmills with their sails merrily twirling a welcome to us.

Ruth and Ben had two children. The elder's name was Lois, she was called 'Little Lois' to distinguish her from Rennie's Aunty Lois. Helen, the other child, was just a baby.

Little Lois was a mischievous tease as we soon found out.

The short honeymoon of two days was soon over and after a good breakfast and a wonderful send off by Aunt Ruth, Uncle Ben and little Lois, we set off for our new home, The White House, Bunkers Hill, North Cray, Sidcup, Kent. This sounded as if it was a manor house, in fact it was an empty farm worker's cottage.

Fortunately we arrived during daylight in high spirits after an easy drive.

It was then we realised some of the disadvantages of our new home. No electric light, but it was fun trimming the oil lamps and filling the primus stove to make our first cup of tea as man and wife at home. It was late December, so night was soon upon us. By the time we had put away clothes and arranged things for the night, we were tired out and so to bed. We managed at first to cook on our primus stove and enjoyed our breakfast. Rennie then tackled the kitchen stove, a monstrous job, but enthusiasm and energy triumphed, and we enjoyed the warmth beginning to infiltrate throughout the cottage. We then found that there was no way of heating water for the bath except by carrying kettles of boiling water. Eventually I managed to clean a five gallon oil drum and fixed it at the head of the bath and using the primus stove managed to heat the bath water on site.

I cannot enumerate the number of essential jobs we had to undertake. There was redecoration of most rooms and make do furnishings, which Rennie charmingly fitted with chintz covers. After our first Christmas we were ready to welcome guests.

At Christmas we visited both sides of the family, so we were not entirely on our own, but of course I had my job to do.

I had no idea what a difficult situation this would be for Rennie. Looking back, she put up with being alone in our cottage, during all the time I spent at hospital and seeing patients in the practice.

Fortunately our first guest was her father, who came to spend a few days with us. I remember he looked askance at the two single beds, but made no comment. Whilst he was with us we visited relatives at Sidcup and that was a reunion for him with his two sisters and brother-in -law.

He returned to Dublin and we went to see him off at Holyhead.

We had let him have the loan of our alarm clock whilst he stayed with us, but after he had gone it was nowhere to be found. As we had only the one alarm, we concluded that he must have packed it in his case absent mindedly. So Rennie wrote to ask if that was what he had done. The reply was prompt and by telegram 'Look inside the other bed'.

There it was! He was marvellous at seeing the amusing side of life, but this particular incident must have assured him that he need have no worries about our marriage. I grew to admire him for the way he tackled the difficulties he had to contend with in Dublin. We tried to convince him that he was always welcome to share our home.

His second marriage was unfortunate.

Rennie's mother must have been an heroic and loving woman.

I regret never having met her. She died when Rennie was seven. She was nearly forty years old and had had four children. Rennie was her third child and the one most like her. Her father adored her and this aroused some discord with her stepmother when her father married again. This early childhood is well portrayed in my wife's autobiography.

Her father had two boys by her stepmother, Joe and Cliff. We shall hear more of them as time passes.

Later on during that first winter we spent some time at my old home at East Dulwich. This was an occasion when Father took his whole family to see the fireworks at the Crystal Palace. Father, when we had settled in our seats, looked at us all and said, "This is a great joy for me, to look around and see all the family." I have never forgotten his expression, nor the emotion in his voice when he fondly regarded us all.

My three brothers were there and my eldest brother's wife, Hetty. It was quite late when we left for our cottage and after driving about halfway in pouring rain, the car broke down and all attempts to restart it failed. We still had about six miles to travel and there was apparently no chance of getting home except by walking. Another motorist saw our dilemma. He stopped, and asked if we would like a lift. Our home was well out of his way, but he insisted on taking us to our front door. This was typical of the fellowship among the motorists at that time. How grateful we both were, and he pooh-poohed our thanks. He had no sooner gone, than my brother Jack arrived in his car.

It was past midnight but he had sensed that we were in trouble.

He had seen our broken down car and realised we needed help.

His foreboding was correct. We have never forgotten his kindness in acting on 'telepathy', when all the chances were that we had got back safely.

After some refreshment in the shape of hot drinks and sandwiches, he returned to his home, whilst we discussed our night of unusual adventures, which included the great kindness of a stranger, followed by my brother's anxiety for our welfare:

The Winter season offered me the chance to try to get our garden in order. There was plenty to do, also we decided to keep some chickens. First we needed a chicken house. So soon after World War I, it was difficult to get wood, so we had to make do with a mass of old newspapers, some galvanised wire netting and wood frames, the four sides and roof were made. The paper was nearly two inches thick and soaked in tar, and soon there was the chicken house ready for habitation, and I may add, very hygienically smelling of tar!.

This makeshift erection lasted for over a year but the hens found the papers interesting and started pecking at the walls until they became more like open-work curtains, and they had to be replaced by a more substantial structure.

Rennie and I decided that we should have a dog so we bought a small puppy, which we christened Pip. He was an intelligent and loyal defender. One day a gypsy called and tried to force Rennie to buy things.

He jammed his foot against the door and became threatening. Rennie called "Pip" and this tiny animal flung himself at the intruder, who fell and then ran off.

A few days later Rennie and Pip were out for a walk, when they saw the gypsy encampment. The gypsies were having a picnic meal. The man who had threatened Rennie scowled angrily at her, so Rennie ordered: "Pip! Stop him!" and Pip flew at the man and scattered the lot, gypsies, food, crockery and created a mild form of havoc.

We were not at all anti-gypsy, but the earlier incident had definitely worried Rennie. I had planted a lot of daffodil bulbs for the spring and when they bloomed they were delightful, but within a day or two we found that they had all been taken. Meanwhile my work went on. We had got our operating table set up and were able to start taking in patients for minor operations. This may have appeared risky, but no operation took place without providing for emergencies.

I was fortunate in being on the staffs of three voluntary hospitals and thus could get help from colleagues in a crisis. We had no trouble, any difficulties were treated as they arose. Christmas 1926, we were due to visit Rennie's sister Eva, who had recently married. Her husband was Sidney Leech, and they lived at Wallington, quite a long journey. The night before our visit there had been a very heavy snowfall and we had to drive along a single track with high banks of snow on each side. At intervals passing bays had been cleared. Being young this was all great fun, but we were relieved to reach the main roadway.

When we returned, a thaw had set in instead of a frost as we feared. A relief to be safe at home!

During the first two years of our tenancy of the White House there was no question of my practising medicine in the area.

During spring and early summer, our home became an irresistible attraction for relatives and friends from Dulwich and King's College Hospital. We were hard put to continue supplying teas to first one lot of visitors and then another. On one Sunday, we had seventeen separate lots to entertain. It was almost a full house that day, as people came and went for hours.

The local farmer and his wife invited us to 'Tea' one day. Fortunately the hour was comparatively late and I was able to get back from hospital in time. I had never experienced such a Gargantuan meal. A plate set in front of me to start with was heaped with food which I managed to eat, certainly at the start with relish, but no sooner had I finished it, than another huge course replaced it. I attempted to do the right thing and enjoy the feast. It was overpowering however, and the next thing I remember was Rennie kicking me under the table. I had fallen asleep and was beginning to snore!

This caused great amusement to the farming fraternity and so I was forgiven.

That summer, Rennie told me she was expecting our first child. This was exciting news indeed. I felt that everyone should know. Rennie assured me that babies had been born before and that there was nothing to worry about!

However the prospect of being a family man was wondrous to me.

I wanted to tell the world, but I was ordered to keep quiet, which was not easy for me.

My Mother was a small woman. Her maiden name was Padley and all her brothers and sisters were of similar stature. I was the only one however to inherit the Padley gene. My brothers were all taller, about five foot ten. There I was five foot six and a half. How I treasured that half inch and I persisted in stretching myself, hoping to achieve five foot seven!

Rennie continued to work hard and, in fact, learnt to ride our motor bicycle right up to the date of the expected arrival of our first-born. No one believed she was pregnant. She had been seen by Professor Gilliat, the senior obstetrician at King's College Hospital, who said that the baby would be a very small child, which was not surprising in view of my ancestry. On St Valentine's Day, the 14th of February 1927, Elizabeth was born. It was a long and exhausting labour. Rennie had developed strong muscles associated with nursing and lifting patients, this condition associated with such a small baby was the probable reason.

A brother practitioner delivered her and Rennie's friend, Nurse Seth-Smith, assisted and stayed with us for the lying-in period. Elizabeth indeed was a small baby, but absolutely beautiful. She had a mass of dark hair and her features were perfect. There had been no 'moulding' during labour. Grandparents, relatives and friends flocked to see the happy mother and her infant.

There could not have been prouder parents, and there could not have been a warmer welcome than the February of that year gave to Mother and Child. It was amazingly spring-like and the temperature was so inviting that when Rennie was up and about we had lunch in the garden. These were halcyon days for our family of three.

Elizabeth was christened by the Rector of the parish church of North Cray; Canon La Touche. Rumour has it 'She winked at him'. Elizabeth was tiny, but so light in weight, that at an early age she was making efforts to walk. This she succeeded in doing at about nine months. Rennie was worried about her small appetite, but of course her needs as regards food were commensurate with her size.

Christmas 1927, was an exciting time for us. Rennie made a tiny skullcap of sparkling silver material and our tiny daughter made her first appearance at our family party, as the Fairy Queen.

We were beginning to fear that she would never grow, and she was so small that she used to run under a small coffee-table and have room to spare. One day, she raced under as usual, but bumped her head slightly. She cried a little and came to us for comfort. She could not understand why we were so pleased in spite of her slight hurt. She had grown!

She had inherited the Padley gene, but though she lacked stature, she developed as a leader.

Our second child was born on October the twenty-seventh, 1928. at a nursing home near King's College Hospital.

She was of average weight and soon began to grow to her sister's height. Rennie had a less distressing labour but this was marred when the ligature on the umbilical cord slipped and our second daughter, Patricia, lost a lot of blood before Rennie realised what was happening. Fortunately her response was in time and she applied quickly a tighter and firm ligature. Patricia was very weak, but thanks to her mother's prompt action, our child, though debilitated at the time, soon improved under her mother's love and care. We both had had a dreadful shock and it must have been far more intense for Rennie. Matron was appalled that such a thing should have happened.

Our lease of the White House was due to expire early in the New Year. We had to think what to do.

****

A week later we returned home, pleased with our now bonny daughter, but in a chastened mood.

We were a happy family. The children thrived and they loved our garden, while our faithful terrier, Pip, seemed to consider himself their guardian.

Soon afterwards my eldest brother, John, and his wife, Mary, came to see us and brought their three children on a visit. The youngest had a cold with a distressing cough. We could hardly believe it, when we heard Mary say: "Kiss the little baby." Before either Rennie or I could intervene, he had done so. Next morning my brother, Jack, rang us up to say that their youngest had whooping cough.

A terrible time befell us, for both our daughters were infected and the illness was virulent.

Unfortunately I had undertaken a locum tenens appointment some miles away. I tried to find a deputy to take my place, but at such short notice that was impossible. Also, the doctor was already away on holiday. This left Rennie to bear the brunt of this ghastly period. I got back as often as I could, and my mother came from Dulwich to bring some comforts and do what she could. The paroxysms seemed to overwhelm our two daughters. Fortunately Rennie had the help of our young maid, Peggy, who was immune, having bad the disease, She helped in every way she could.

My mother was appalled at Rennie's plight, especially as I was away so much doing this locum. At her age, she had packed as much as she could carry and set out by public transport, and had to walk from Bexley Station, (as there was no taxi), all the way from Bexley Station to North Cray.

Rennie's compassionate heart was overwhelmed at this thoughtful and loving aid by my mother, and it created a lasting bond between them.

My locum was a short one but seemed endless at the time. In a few weeks the children, though still weak, were slowly regaining their strength, and thankfully we were able to resume our normal lives.

A few weeks later, I was seeing patients at the old home in East Dulwich when Jack's wife, Mary, asked me to call in to see their children, especially the eldest, David, then about seven. He was suffering from earache.

I examined him carefully and was startled at what I found. He had all the transient warning signs of incipient bacterial meningitis due to infection of the middle ear.

This in the days before antibiotics meant that he should be admitted to hospital at once as an emergency. I wanted to arrange his admission to King's College Hospital at once. Mary insisted that she would wait until Jack had returned. Later he rang up to say all the signs I had quoted were not present. David had a good appetite and after supper was now fast asleep.

Those ominous signs were unheeded with disbelief.

Jack was a senior clinician and had won a gold medical for his brilliance. I think that he was mentally unable to accept that his son might be in mortal danger and that I might conceivably be correct.

The next morning, about eighteen hours after I had seen my nephew, poor David was in the agonising throes of acute bacterial meningitis. He was rushed to hospital, operated on at once, but it was too late, and in a few days my nephew, a child of promise, had died.

Meanwhile his younger brother, Beverly, had shown similar symptoms and he was operated on at once. His recovery was long and anxious, but he survived.

This added to the already depressed and fearful anxiety of Rennie and myself as to what further disaster might befall. Then one morning I found 'Pip' lying dead in the garden. He had apparently been poisoned.

Was this sad event the Gypsy's revenge?

By now the lease of the White House was nearly at the end.

Rennie and I wondered what we should do. Our present home with its large garden, lawns, and orchard, still held memories which were precious to us, though recent so sad events had had their own effect.

What should we decide to do?

For Elizabeth Pip's death was her first experience of mortality. Her grief was pitiful to see and we arranged a quiet little funeral ceremony for him as a mark of our love and gratitude for his canine loyalty and devotion. Elizabeth marked his grave with a special stone.

Patricia was still only just emerging from babyhood, so this sad event meant nothing to her.

My Mother was still with us and was to share our new home. My Father had died the year Elizabeth was born. Rennie nursed him during his last days at the old home on The Rye. He suffered terribly from "air hunger" which Rennie eased with oxygen, and comforted him as far as she possibly could. It was sad that he died before Elizabeth was born, because he had been looking forward to the birth of his new grandchild. For my mother, Rennie's unselfish and compassionate presence must have seemed an answer to her prayers.

Rennie was present to hear Father's dramatic last words.

During his younger days he had been a keen fly fisherman and he seemed to go back to his youth. He raised himself up and made an imaginary cast with a fly-fishing rod, then apparently caught a fish, and exclaimed with triumph "What a whopper!" These were his final words and he died with a look of joy on his face.

Mother's presence and help at the White House during the children's terrible attack of whooping cough were an expression of her admiration and love for her daughter-in-law. In 1929 our lease was in its last days. We had to decide what to do.

This difficulty was resolved for us in a most unexpected way.

In 1926, the Irish Constitution was changed by President De Valera from "The Irish Free State" to "The Republic of Ireland."

This created what seemed an insoluble problem. How could a "Republic" form part of "The British Empire"?

The British Empire was still almost intact, and it seemed impossible for a republic to acknowledge a monarch as the titular head. Later, the granting of independence to India, Pakistan, Nigeria and other countries, led to the change of title from "Empire" to "Commonwealth."

Many of the Irish population, who were loyal to the idea of a united nation of the British Isles, (both Roman Catholic and Protestant), decided to leave the Republic and find new homes in other parts of the kingdom. Most came to England, among them the Countess of Limerick, her personal friends, and Dr. Herd and his wife. They settled in Bexley, Kent. The countess purchased the hall, once the home of "The Fair Maid of Kent." Dr. Herd bought a general medical practice in Bexley, and became a popular member of the community.

Unfortunately, his health was not good, so he asked me to help him, and, as his condition worsened, I acted as his locum. He realised that his condition was grave and he asked me if I would like to purchase his house and practice.

This fortunate offer was made just as the lease of The White House was nearly up. I gladly accepted his proposition, and soon afterwards, to our sorrow, our friend and benefactor, Dr. Herd, died.

When Dr. Herd died, I opened a surgery in Bexley High Street to continue his general practice.

At this time we moved from the White House to Grangehurst, Hurst Road, Bexley; Dr. Herd's old residence.

This was a large family house situated in lovely grounds. The front garden had two entrances, with a lawn and central bed of azaleas. There were two tennis courts, an orchard, two lawns, a garage, (room for more than two cars), a large outbuilding, and a garden shed.

The rooms in the house were spacious indeed compared with our first home! Grangehurst had a large dining room - which was large enough for a dance - the drawing room opened out into a charming bell shaped conservatory.

The kitchen was huge, with both scullery and pantry.

The first floor had four large bedrooms, a super bathroom with a shower, which was in an alcove at the head of the bath. When turned on, numerous sprays of water covered one from head to foot!

The second floor had three attics, two large and one small. Our furniture from the White House was almost lost in such an expanse.

Rennie was amazing with, it seemed to me, tireless energy. She made curtains for every window, and soon created a home for all the family. Her success in such a short time was miraculous.

My mother helped by sending furniture from Rye.

Later Mother left the Rye, and shared part of our new home. She brought with her 'the old family cook', who was able to help Rennie, or rather, 'share', some of the household tasks. There were a number of problems for us to solve. The most difficult was financial. Until now we had steered clear of running into debt to any large extent.

Buying this house, and the late Dr. Herd's practice involved obtaining a mortgage, and insurance to cover illness etc. This period was a presage of the present day financial difficulties. The worldwide recession of the thirties was about to occur.

Nevertheless the practice increased, Grangehurst in effect became a great help as Rennie used her nursing skills to the full. Numbers of relations, friends, and patients, came to Grangehurst; some to have babies, others for operations. Meanwhile the two children were growing. Soon there would be schooling to consider. Elizabeth was nearly five when one summer day she was not to be found. We searched all likely places, inside the house and all over the garden. Should we tell the police?

Then we heard her high child's voice calling

"You can't find me!"

Finally we saw her. She was high up an apple tree, hanging upside down with her legs over a branch! Rennie and I wondered how to get her down, but we need not have worried, for she climbed down as lightly as a mischievous monkey. Rennie told her never to frighten us again like that, which she promised, and so all was well once more.

This was the time of the pageants, and the euphoria, which was beginning to lessen.

One morning during surgery hours, a well dressed middle aged woman called as the last patient left.

"Doctor," she said,

"I am not a patient but a qualified midwife and trained nurse. My name is Marks, Miss Marks, and I would value your advice. I propose to start a Nursing Home in Bexley, and I would appreciate your help. I have already approached the other doctors in the area, and they have approved."

At first my heart sank. This would be in competition with Grangehurst. On second thought, I realised what a great advantage such a Nursing Home could be. The more details she gave me, the more interested I became.

I asked if she would have an operating theatre. She replied that there was a room which could be adapted. I offered my help in providing the operating table and certain other surgical articles that I had.

Miss Marks told me she would have other trained nurses and assistant staff as required.

I became not only interested but enthusiastic. What a blessing this would be for Rennie! It would relieve her from being disturbed at night, and from endless other nursing chores. So Elmhurst Nursing and Maternity Home became a reality, much to the benefit of Bexley and area residents, and may I add, to Rennie and myself.

My colleagues at the Sydenham Children's Hospital and elsewhere were interested and provided specialist help.

One day as evening surgery was coming to an end, I had an emergency call to the Children's Hospital at Sydenham. I had hoped to get home earlier than usual, but off I had to go. Fortunately the emergency turned out to be minor, and I soon left for home.

My car was a Humber-Snipe and it seemed to purr sweetly along. There was little traffic at the time and I kept as far as possible to the centre of the road to avoid any potholes near the verge. I had only a mile or two further to go when I reached the village of Bridgen. It was just after closing time when the Inn door opened, as mine host rather unsteadily let his Alsatian sheepdog out. The dog dashed straight across the road. To avoid hitting the animal I braked sharply and pulled over to the nearside verge. There was a loud thump as the car bounced to a stop.

Carefully, I opened the car door and got out to see what had happened. I was confronted by the irate innkeeper. He was too far 'gone' to recognise me and shouted

"You bl--dy murderer! You deserve to be hanged. You're not fit to push a pram, let alone drive a car. If I had my way you'd be jailed for life!"

Having warmed up with these few words, he proceeded to pass doubts as to my ancestors, characters of which he gave a far from complimentary opinion. He then paused to regain his breath.

By this time the street was filled with local folk, who were enjoying every minute. I took advantage of his pause to say

"When you have finished describing me, I'll tell you what I what I think of you."

This remark started a further torrent of abuse and ended with,

"If I had a halter to hand, I'd hang you myself!"

Mindful of the saying 'A soft answer turneth away wrath', I said "I think you are very rude."

This comment brought loud laughter from the crowd, whether at me or my tormentor is anyone's guess.

At this precise moment the sheepdog came bounding back in high spirits. He looked around and appeared to sum up the situation. Then he sat down on his haunches, stretched his neck and uttered howl after howl! Was he laughing? This started us all off; the innkeeper, who by now had recognised me (rather shamefacedly), the locals, and me.

'Laughter is the best medicine', is the saying. It certainly was in this case.

After being in Bexley a few years, most of the publicans were patients. I was a teetotaller!

Though small at that time, the town was a busy one. There were local societies such as the Women's Institute, the Dramatic Society, and sports clubs, and of course the Boy Scouts and Girl Guides.

The Volunteer Fire Brigade was of exceptional efficiency. The alarm was sounded by firing off one of the First World War mortar shells, (the original air raid warning).

On one occasion the fire engine arrived at the scene of the fire just as the mortar shell gave the warning. The members had all been alerted by telephone before firing off the mortar shell!

The Bexley practice increased and included a residential estate, Baldwyns Park, which adjoined Joydens Wood. Joydens Wood in particular was the home of some eccentric characters. One was a 'busker' who was a familiar and popular figure at the theatre queues in the West End. I was asked to see him as he was suffering from an attack of influenza.

His wooden hut (it could not be described as a bungalow) was in the depths of the wood.

When I reached his front door, I heard a voice from within say "Come in, doctor."

I remember being reminded of 'Little Red Riding Hood' when she heard "Lift up the latch and the bobbin will fall." She could not have been more taken aback at what she saw than I was at what awaited me.

My patient was in a four-poster bed which took up most of the room, but what took my breath away was that there were birds everywhere. They were roosting on every available perch, both top and bottom of the bedposts, those less fortunate had to perch on other articles of furniture. I cannot describe the atmosphere other than 'avian' to the Nth. degree.

They were wild birds, mostly jackdaws, and my patient possessed an intimate understanding of, and affection for them. I believe they appreciated this to the full. He must have developed some degree of immunity from avian diseases.

My patient soon recovered and resumed his trips to the theatre queues. The jackdaws would choose silver rather than copper coins to drop into his cap amid admiring spectators. He was to be seen up to the time of the second world war and there must be many people today who can remember him. Later, I believe, the local health authority took exception to his living conditions, but by then he was a very old man.

Before my time, Sir Hugh Bessemer, the steel magnate, lived in the Baldwyns - Joydens Wood area, and he was the first man to build and fly a heavier than air aeroplane. This plane was propeller driven by a steam engine which was powerful enough, in spite of the weight factor to succeed in getting the craft airborne.

The trial flight took place where space was limited. So a runway was built with rails, and the plane had a connecting line so as to control the landing. The aircraft took off and flew successfully, but landing proved something of a disaster. The plane was damaged beyond repair. Fortunately the engine was salvaged, and it is now in the Science Museum. The flight is not officially recognised as it was not 'free'. So it is, that Wilbur Wright holds the distinction of being the first man 'to fly free'.

Late one evening I had an urgent call to Joydens Wood to a maternity case. The expectant mother was not a patient of mine, but the midwife concerned was out on another case. It was a moonless night, but I knew the locality and was soon on the doorstep.

The front door was ajar, and so after knocking to introduce myself I entered the bungalow. I have never seen a tidier room in connection with an urgent maternity case.

"It's all over, Doctor," exclaimed the smiling mother sitting up in her bed.

"It all happened so quickly that I thought it best not to wait for you or the nurse. Look isn't he a lovely baby? I've cleaned up everything and tied and cut the cord."

It had certainly been a precipitate labour and the child was the recent addition to a numerous family of others who were fast asleep.

I was wondering whether her previous experiences of giving birth had been as speedy, when there came a knock at the door which I had closed behind me.

"That'll be nurse, I expect" beamed the fond mother, who seemed to think it was all a huge joke.

I opened the front door and saw only pitch black darkness except for a few bright stars.

Then I heard someone giggling about roundabout knee level. There were two steps up to the threshold. I looked down and glimpsed a pair of bright eyes laughing at me.

"It's lil-ole Nurse Jackson, Doctor!" said a blithe voice. She stepped into the room. I still could not at first believe that what I beheld wasn't some benign fairy. My height is only five foot and six inches, but the dainty figure before me only reached to my shoulders. She was a negress and she positively sparkled with 'joie de vivre'.

Bursting with energy, she bustled about chatting merrily to the mother and cooing indulgently over the baby.

She was a certified midwife and loved by the woodlanders.

One day when I arrived for morning surgery at the High Street, I was surprised to see, sitting in a deck-chair on the front lawn, a patient from Joydens Wood. She had a small table, a book and Thermos flask, and appeared to be well established there.

She greeted me with glee, saying "I was determined to be your first patient this morning."

I could not help but feel there was something magical about Joydens Wood, which had a unique effect on its inhabitants.

One of the patients, who came to Bexley with Dr. Herd, had been desperately ill with breast cancer and was now convalescent after an operation and X-ray treatment. She was an ardent Protestant loyalist, a great friend of the Countess of Limerick, and had her full share of Irish blarney. I hoped one day to outdo her flattery. The chance came when she asked for a special appointment. In due course as I entered the room, she exclaimed,

"Dr. Robinson, when you enter a room, it is like a ray of sunshine."

"Madam," I replied "I am but a feeble mirror."

She enjoyed several more years of life, but eventually succumbed to the dreaded disease.

The telephone rang shrilly one day, the call was from Hall Place, the Countess of Limerick has had an accident. Please call urgently.

Please visit at once.

The Countess was another ardent Protestant and was an active campaigner for her faith. She had a habit of sending for young girls from Ireland to train as maids.

If they were Roman Catholics, the countess would zealously attempt to convert them to what she believed to be the true faith.

She had some successes, but one maid must have written home or told the local priest. For the maid tried to convert her mistress, with predictable results! The countess was furious and the maid was dismissed. I do not know the exact details, as to whether it was the maid, or the countess, who slammed the front door, as she exhorted "Never darken my doors again."

When I arrived, the countess was sitting up in a huge double bed with a cold compress on her head secured by a white linen sling from her chin, tied in a bow on top.

She explained how the accident happened,

"It was all the fault of that ungrateful maid. I told her never to darken my doors again, then the front door slammed behind her and the fanlight fell down on my head!"

There had been a considerable haemorrhage from the superficial scalp wound. After cleansing I closed the cut under local anaesthesia, and soon the countess was her buoyant self again. Her huge unusual double bed now drew my attention. I had to ask about it. This request temporarily helped her forget her mishap as, full of enthusiasm, she described how the bed had come into her family's possession.

During the flight of the Spanish Armada along the west coast of Ireland, one of the galleons was driven ashore and wrecked.

The bed was salvaged in good condition.

Along the back was a series of shelves and small cupboards. Originally these contained a Holy Bible, a pair of loaded pistols, writing materials, and charts.

I was to see this bed again in the future but that occasion was to be years ahead.

****

Our summer holidays were always difficult to arrange and expenses had to be cut to the minimum, especially as a locum tenens had to be paid. Yet we had some wonderful times caravanning in the South West or Wales. Rennie loved the Welsh countryside and especially Anglesey with its Celtic traditions and archaeological treasures.

One year there was almost an epidemic of virulent acute otitis media, especially among young children. Apart from the extra visiting this entailed in the practice, hospital admissions for acute mastoiditis and broncho-pneumonia filled all childrens' hospital beds to overflowing.

One week the number of emergency operations at The South Eastern Hospital was so great that I had no sleep for three nights. The stocks of sterilised towels at the hospital became exhausted and more had to be sent for from London. Eventually even this supply ran out and I used clean towels soaked in strong antiseptic lotion.

At last the strain began to ease and I had at least two nights sleep at home, when the telephone rang from the hospital.

The medical paediatrician at the hospital asked me to see a child patient of his who had broncho-pneumonia, associated with a postnasal discharge. He was not present when I arrived. On examining this child, who was about eighteen months old, I could see the muco-pus poring down from the back of her nose. Then I looked at her ears. They were both inflamed, and the mastoid areas were both swollen, tender and spongy to the touch.

I decided that urgent opening of each mastoid was the only hope of saving the child's life. I had just exposed the mastoid bone on one side, when the physician burst into the theatre and ordered:-

"Stop, the child will never stand an operation."

He was too late, for with a small steel spoon I had scooped out infected spongy bone and exposed the source of infection on one side, and rapidly repeated the operation on the other side. The child was returned to the ward and a change was soon evident. The tearing, exhausting and strident coughing ceased and was followed by peaceful sleep. Her temperature soon dropped to normal and full recovery followed.

Today such a condition is unlikely to develop for with the discovery of penicillin and other antibiotics the infection would be eradicated in the early stage.

The hospital routine had returned to normal, (if that description is appropriate) when I had another emergency call, a case of extreme urgency.

This child presented all the alarming symptoms of meningeal irritation and an immediate mastoid operation was necessary.

The mother refused to authorise the operation as her husband was a Plymouth brother. Every minute was precious if the child was to have any chance of recovery. I pointed out that only poisoned blood would be removed, certainly not 'spilt'. I had either to see this child endure the fate of my late nephew, or risk operating without permission.

Fortunately the sad tale of my nephew's death convinced the mother, and she signed the needed form of authority. The theatre staff and the anaesthetist were waiting, so the operation was done at once. I hoped it was not too late. It went well and once over, I hoped the prognosis would be good.

When I reached the hospital entrance hall, a man strode up to me and demanded

"Are you Mr. Robinson?"

"Yes," I replied.

"Have you operated on my daughter?" he challenged me, red in the face.

"Yes," I faltered, suddenly alarmed.

He was a powerful man and the next thing I knew I was sailing down the hospital front steps with the loss of two teeth.

He was restrained by the hospital staff, whilst his distressed tear-stained wife looked on.

Did I wish to charge him with assault? I was asked. I could see no point in that, as I looked at the frantic fanatic, who was obviously regretting his hasty action.

Mercifully the child recovered, left hospital, and I never saw either the child or the parents again.

These few weeks had not been good for the practice, as apart from the difficulty of attending surgeries, I was so fatigued that one day I fell asleep during a visit.

Then, inevitably I suppose, I became ill myself.

One day, whilst walking up a slight hill, I was forced to ask Rennie to slow down, as I was out of breath.

Next morning I had a definite right maxillary (cheek bone) sinusitis.

I saw my old chief at King's College Hospital, Mr. Hope, Honorary Ear Nose and Throat surgeon. He admitted me there and then for further investigation. Next morning I had a painful big toe and jokes were made about 'gout'. Next day I developed acute polyarticular arthritis and acute myocarditis, (inflammation of the heart). The cardiologist felt that as I had developed "heart block", there was little hope of my recovery and advised Rennie to sell the practice before it became a death vacancy.

Rennie would not hear of that, but courageously took in resident patients, looked after our children and managed to visit me in hospital.

Obviously I recovered sufficiently to return home. It was twelve months before I was able to close my hands enough to hold an instrument, or even a spoon, for long. During this period, my brother, Oliver, drove down to Bexley to do what he could to hold the practice together.

Fortunately I had a sickness and life insurance, which helped. Meantime, Rennie took in patients who required constant supervision as they were mentally subnormal. One of them had her own full time nurse companion.

At last, after almost another six months, it seemed that overnight my stiffness disappeared, and I rapidly recovered. Then came the reckoning. Financially we were in difficulty. Grangehurst was far too expensive and had to go.

We moved to the surgery which was a house built several centuries ago, and which had a charm of its own. Rennie made a four poster bed. She got me to make the posts and then sewed the hangings, and the result was in tune with the old beams and the period room.

My account at the bank was in a parlous state and one day the bank manager sent for me. He showed me a scheme by a financial firm, who were prepared to purchase the practice which I would continue to run as their employee.

I asked what security would I have if they decided to sell the practice over my head? The answer, when all 'ifs and buts' were taken into account, was none.

Miss Marks, matron of the nursing home, who was by now a family friend, when she heard of our difficulty, asked how much the debt at the bank was.

I told her and she promptly wrote out a cheque for the full amount. I had to compel her to accept interest on this generous offer. Thankfully I cleared the overdraft. This was indeed a happy issue out of our financial impasse.

The bank manager was a patient, and I was startled when, soon afterwards, he rang up in a panic to say that he had been going over accounts, and found that mine was still heavily overdrawn. He must see me before his branch's quarterly report was sent in to head office. Would I please come as soon as possible? Rennie and I were horrified and we sped to the bank at top speed.

There we were met by a smiling manager, who said:

"I am sorry if I alarmed you, but I had put a decimal point in the wrong place, your account is in credit."

What a relief, but his credit, as a bank manager, dropped a few points.

One of my patients was a man in middle age, who suffered from a spinal deformity which had developed gradually. As a result, he stooped almost at a right angle and used a stick to support himself when walking. He was a character, and used to go regularly to the Windmill Theatre, whose slogan was that it never closed. Its programme was one of exotic choral dancing. He would arrive early and stay as long as possible, sometimes seeing the same programme over and over again.

He would then write to the producer, criticising erotic or provocative saucy scenes, which he had lapped up. The manager asked him to call to see him.

This my patient did and he was cordially received and shown round. He saw at first hand the professional talent and ingenuity which went into each programme. He greatly enjoyed all of this, especially meeting some of the attractive dancers. The producer explained that his criticisms were most helpful and he wondered if perhaps my patient would like to take a financial interest and invest some capital in the production. This proposal did not appeal to my patient at all.

He was a Scotsman and indeed 'canny', as well as eccentric.

His wife, too had her foibles.

She was a tornado at croquet, carrying all before her at lightening speed to end victorious, leaving her late opponents busily retrieving their scattered balls.

They were a pair of oddities who did much to enliven our social life. Needless to say my patient made no investment in the theatre, especially as his back was giving him so much discomfort.

Eventually, he agreed to see an orthopaedic surgeon, after putting it off as long as he could.

The consultant, after studying my patient's x-ray films, advised manipulation under general anaesthesia.

Surprisingly, he agreed and he was admitted to the nursing home.

The manipulation was a success, but the result was that instead a stance resembling a bent pin, he was as perpendicular as a flagpole. He became known in Bexley as the walking miracle. I visited him just before he left the nursing home,

"Are you going home ?" he asked me.

"Yes" I said.

It so happened that my car was being serviced and I had walked.

"I've ordered a taxi," he went on. "Will you come back with me?"

"Thank you" I replied, grateful for the offer.

"Good," he said with a gleam in his eye, "The cost of the taxi is one pound, so that will be ten shillings each!"

I might have known it wasn't a free gift.

Rennie and I had noticed that our younger daughter, Paddy, was tiring easily and tended to limp. We decided to ask the orthopaedic surgeon to see her.

He examined her with great care and found that one leg was slightly shorter than the other.

Paddy endured all the examination and walked up and down when told without a murmur. Mr. Carlton, the orthopaedic surgeon, ordered special boots for her. The one for the shorter leg was built up, to give an equal level for standing or walking. Paddy to all appearances, placidly put up with all this and with wearing the boots. Inwardly she must have hated to feel different from her friends. Sensing her consciousness of it 'they began to pick on' her in various ways.

We of course were unaware of her problems. She never

complained but must have bottled up her resentment.

If only we had realised this, we could have helped her through this difficult time. Her posture improved, and she tired less easily, which was physically good, but she had to be watched in order to avoid any curvature of the spine 'scoliosis'. Throughout this period her good nature showed itself when she would try to take the blame for any mishap whilst playing with others.

When we moved to the High Street, my Mother left Bexley and rented a flat near Denmark Hill within reasonable distance of her old home and her circle of family friends. She was pleased to be near St. Matthew's church, Denmark Hill, close to King's College Hospital.

We could take the two girls with us sometimes on weekend visits, and they have happy memories of her.

This was in the early thirties, when, although the optimism following the end of World War I was ebbing, private housing was going ahead with remarkable speed.

A leading example was the "Ideal Homes" company. I remember watching them building housing estates near Bexley. The bricklayers, carpenters and other skilled craftsmen, with their assistants, worked with amazing rapidity. I wondered whether they were paid at performance rates.

A two bedroom house, with all conveniences, would cost from £250 to £350, depending on whether it was a terrace house, semi-detached or standing on its own ground. Many people referred to them as 'jerry built' and added that they had no prospect of long life.

Nevertheless they are still much sought after and are now valued at about one hundred times the original price! I bought two, each in different areas as branches of the practice.

Meantime in Germany, Hitler was increasing his following, but few people realised the extent of his ambition. Apart from Germany, there were similar signs of political unrest in Italy and Spain.

****

1933 was a fateful year for our family.

The practice was increasing and with the start of the London Public Medical Service, another regular quarterly cheque was paid to the patient's doctor. The Public Medical Service was not a government service, but a similar scheme by which dependants of a National Insured person could cover his or her dependants for twopence a week.

This was a great step forward for those few 'panel' patients, who could not afford private fees for their dependants. Previously these dependants were treated without charge. As the financial side of the practice improved, I decided to buy another car, turning in my ancient vehicle in part exchange. After my earlier experience, I decided against any instalment system and paid outright. The car was a Morris-Oxford about two years old and in first class condition. I transferred the insurance policy, which was third party, fire and theft only. I decided to change to full cover as soon as finances permitted. This turned out to be a foolish economy.

Two days after the purchase, I was driving on a main road when a motor cyclist, with a pillion passenger travelling at a fast speed, tried to turn into the main road. I stopped at once, but another car coming towards me prevented the motor cyclist turning right, he tried to stop but skidded and crashed straight into the bonnet of my car.

The pillion passenger was flung high into the air over my vehicle, and landed in a sitting position behind it. The driver was hurled, face down, across the bonnet of my car.

The suddenness of this catastrophe seemed unbelievable. I saw the body across the car's bonnet and a part of his face was turned towards me. It was purple and getting denser and darker. I seized my bag, and leapt from the car. Death from asphyxia, if not already a fact, was imminent. I lifted the inert body off the bonnet and laid it on the pavement. Then I opened my emergency bag and fortunately I managed to get a gag between his teeth and opened his mouth. His tongue was blocking the airway. With tongue forceps I pulled the tongue clear and with a gasp he took a breath of air. He was still unconscious but breathing, and his colour was improving. This gave me enough respite to look at the other casualty. He was also unconscious but breathing. By now other people began to collect and I was able to send for the ambulance, which arrived quickly and took both casualties to hospital. Both recovered and eventually returned home.

My car was wrecked as regards road worthiness. The motorcycle was wedged into the front of the car, smashing the radiator and both front ends of the chassis were bent inwards gripping the motorbicycle. This was the first case of 'joy riding' I had heard of, so prevalent today. The motorbicycle had been stolen and the insurance void as the culprits were young boys. The wrecked Morris-Oxford fetched enough money for me to buy back the car I had sold as part exchange!

This misfortune was later to be followed by an autumn tragedy. Meantime summer was in full bloom and the whole family was looking forward to a seaside holiday in our caravan.

We went to the south coast and camped at Climping near Arundel. The children enjoyed the picnics and fun on the beach.

One day we decided to visit Arundel and were very impressed by the castle. Then we decided to see the interior of St. Nichola's church. Rennie and I, with our two young girls, entered the church, and were walking down the centre aisle, when an agitated nun appeared and indignantly requested us to take the two girls out of the church, as their heads were uncovered. This demand seemed so unreasonable to me that I was taken aback and felt quite shocked. Then I thought of Christ's words and said,

"Jesus remarked - Suffer the little children to come unto me and forbid them not."

Her whole attitude changed and she murmured,

"Please wait."

She hurried off and soon returned with two cloths, to place on their heads. It was then our turn to confess to our ignorance and so this episode ended with mutual understanding.

We had a small sailing dinghy and we went for a sailing trip from Arundel down the river on the ebbtide. We had with us my nephew, Beverley, who then was about twelve. All went well until we returned, when the tide was coming in. As we neared the bridge over the river I dropped anchor, and started to take down the mast, to avoid catching the top against the bridge. An onlooker leant over the parapet and shouted,

"There's no need to unstep the mast, from here I can see you've plenty of clearance, at least two feet."

I accepted his assurance, and pulled up the anchor.

At once the current swept the dinghy towards the bridge.

Before I could do anything to avoid it, the tip of the mast caught on the parapet of the bridge, the dinghy turned broadside on to the current and was in imminent danger of capsizing.

I yelled to Beverley, "Jump forward," which, thank heavens, he did with alacrity. This depressed the bow, and the mast just cleared. A disaster had narrowly been avoided, and of course our voluntary adviser had taken himself off.

Since then, when faced with advice different from my own opinion in an emergency, I choose the safer way, whichever that might be.

Soon after we had returned home, Rennie told me she hoped she was expecting another baby. If so, the child would be born the following March.

We decided not to tell my mother until we were certain. Mother and her great friend, Miss Garland, were members of St. Matthew's church parochial council and were keen workers. They attended church meetings regularly, and their joint efforts were much in demand and greatly appreciated.

On Saturday, September the 30th 1933, Mother and Miss Garland had been to a meeting of the church council and were returning home. It was already dusk as they stepped off the pavement, into the road to cross Denmark Hill.

A car without lights, travelling at approximately forty five miles an hour, knocked them both down and did not stop, although the passenger in the car shouted to the driver, "Stop you have knocked down a woman"!

My poor Mother must have been killed instantly.

Miss Garland was unconscious, had multiple compound fractures and severe internal injuries. She died the following morning. The car was eventually stopped at Camberwell Green by a tram driver, who told the motorist that there was a woman's handbag hanging on the handle of his door and that grey hairs were stuck onto the front bumper of his car.

At the inquest the case was adjourned. In the words of the coroner, "I will make no further observation at this stage, except to inform you that the case is one which may assume a grave aspect."

Later, a charge of manslaughter was brought against the driver, but the defence counsel claimed that it was another car which had knocked down the two women and the accused had been unable to avoid the two casualties.

His plea was accepted, although no other vehicle had been mentioned at the earlier inquiry.

However that may have been, my Mother and her great friend had left their place of worship to walk into the presence of the Almighty.

One of our most poignant regrets was that she had not known that we were hoping for another baby in the Spring.

The children sadly missed their 'Ga-Ga', as they had fondly called her, and have always so remembered her.

Mother was mourned not only by her family and friends but also by her audiences which she had entertained in the past.

Soon after my mother's death I called at the old family house on the Rye to discuss the future with my elder brother, Oliver. I had come by train and I was walking back to catch the bus for the station, when I saw coming towards me one of the brother officers who had been in the Middlesex regiment with me in 1916, at the time of my downfall during the field-day at Colchester, prior to embarkation for France. I was amazed to see him, as the unit had suffered dreadful casualties on hill 60 which the German sappers had undermined and then blown up. He had not apparently recognised me, so I stopped him to ask if he was in the Middlesex regiment in 1916. Yes, he replied, he had been. I held out my hand and said how pleased I was to meet him again. He glanced at my hand, then at my face and said "Good-day to you, Sir," and walked away.

This was due of course to the imputation that I had 'dodged the column'. I have mentioned this incident because it probably had a big influence on me when the Second World War broke out. My friend, Gerald Rudolf, had a similar experience. He was a far from fit man, and was not graded 'Al'. So he started his medical training with me during World War One.

When that war ended, returning troops were apt to despise anyone who, in their view, had dodged the column.

On St. George's day, the 23rd of April, 1934, our third child was born. The baby was a boy to the joy of all the family; our two daughters, now aged six and four, had longed for a baby brother.

****

The day before his birth, I had left for hospital, when Rennie realised that labour had started.

My wife had already taken the girls to school in her car, so rather than wait for a taxi she drove herself to the nursing home, much to the surprise of Miss Marks, who had never known of a woman in labour driving herself to hospital.

Rennie had a less difficult labour, and was delighted that her baby was a boy, after having the two girls. He was very like his mother and full of vigour.

He was christened Waring Robinson, in memory of his paternal grandfather and his loving wife, my mother, so recently taken from the family.

The lying-in period soon passed and Rennie and babe were welcomed home with joy and thankfulness.

The High Street house was too small for our family of five, and so, whilst it continued as the main centre of the practice for the time being, I decided to look for a larger home.

Fortunately, an excellent opportunity arose in Parkhill Road, Bexley. The house was opposite St. John's church and its name was St. Laurence.

It was not quite as lavish as Grangehurst, but it had a large front garden, no garage, but an extensive garden with fruit trees at the back.

The interior contained two reception rooms, the one opening into the other, ideal for entertainments, children's plays, or charades. The dining room had a service hatch opening into a first class kitchen, upstairs five bedrooms added appeal.

A housing mortgage was arranged and we moved into our new home. Rennie was faced with making St. Laurence her own family home. She set about this with her boundless enthusiasm and harmoniously attractive sense of colour. There were so many variations in the juxtapositioning of articles of furniture, that I arrived home to one change of surroundings after another until the final pleasing arrangement.

Busy as Rennie was with all this, she found time to start a welfare clinic for mothers and young children at the branch surgery at Carisbrooke Avenue, Bexley.

Each of the branch surgeries had a resident caretaker family, who helped to make this scheme a success.

Soon after we had all settled in at St. Laurence, I had a telephone request from the Matron of the nursing home. Would I attend a maternity case? The baby was due in a few months. The case was that of a young single girl. All expenses were to be paid by the father-to-be, or the future grandfather-to-be, I had no idea which. The only stipulation was that a doctor and a midwife should both be present at the birth.

I accepted the offer, after reassurance that the mother-to-be would receive adequate ante-natal care prior to her admission to the home. She arrived about two weeks before the expected date. This enabled the pre-natal examinations, general health, position of the baby, and its condition, to be determined well in advance. Another maternity case was admitted with early labour pains at about the same time as my case was due. She was not one of my patients.

My patient started in labour and I received the expected call. When I arrived at the home, she was definitely in labour.

Although it was a first baby, with such a young woman everything pointed to an early delivery.

From the comings and goings I gathered that the other woman was at the same stage. Within twenty four hours of the commencement of the 'breaking of the waters' my patient had a lusty boy. I was thinking what a happy start in life it would have been for her if she had been married, when the baby was spirited out of the room before it was seen by its mother. Matron must have guessed my thoughts, for she told me the mother had agreed to this, and please would I not remark about it.

The sequel astonished me. It concerned the other 'maternity' case.

In spite of her baby's disappearance, the young mother made a quick recovery from her ordeal. Yet I felt such a denial of her natural maternal love would inevitably leave a conscious or subconscious, feeling of culpability.

I have no idea whether she had any knowledge of her child's possible future.

This lay with the other 'maternity' admission. She was nearing the age when all hope of having a child was fast disappearing. Her husband's family were landed gentry and he was desperately anxious for a male heir. For years, the couple's hopes of a child had come to nothing. The wife suggested adoption, but to her husband such an idea was out of the question.

Her marriage was subjected to intolerable strain.

She knew the matron of the home, and driven by the fear that if she failed to produce an heir her marriage might break down, she consulted Matron, and they decided that if a young single woman sought help in her distress, she could be admitted to the home and the child adopted.

Knowing her husband's intolerant view of adoption, the wife decided that if such an opportunity arose and the pregnancy was in an early stage, she would tell her husband that at last she was pregnant.

As soon as she heard from the matron that a young girl of good family was 'in trouble', and was to be admitted to the home in due course, she put her plan into operation.

She suggested that she would sleep on her own for the time being in order to enhance the hope of a healthy pregnancy. Her husband, who was only too anxious for an heir, readily agreed. So she slept on her own, and padded herself out as the weeks passed. Finally she entered the home as a 'maternity case'. When my patient had recovered sufficiently, I was leaving the home, when the husband of the other woman burst excitedly in. I had never met him, but he almost shouted to me with such triumph in his voice. "I have just registered the birth of my heir and I have entered him for my old school!"

This was one of the most elite public schools of the country. I was so carried away by his enthusiasm, that I found myself shaking him by the hand and rejoicing with him. He grasped me with both hands and insisted

"Come in to meet my wife and heir."

There they were, the wife cradling the babe, tears of joy in her eyes, and her adoring husband, his ambition of an heir fulfilled.

In my opinion there could be no point in exposing the deception. To do so would be not only to humiliate all three of that family, it would also destroy the trust between Matron and myself, and deprive a changeling of a superb start in life. These were the momentary thoughts that flashed through my mind as I gazed at the trio.

Two wrongs cannot make one right, it is said, but these three must surely be right for the future.

That all happened nearly sixty years ago.

How they eventually fared, I have no idea. To make any attempt to find out would be unwise and perhaps disastrous.

The matron adopted two other changelings herself. One was a girl who was coloured, the other was a boy. They both married and now have children of their own.

Matron died shortly after the end of World War Two, all who knew her, as friends or professionally, regretted her passing. Curiously enough, her death is linked in my mind with the end of the Voluntary Hospital Service and the advent of the National Health Hospital Service.

With the former freedom of action by the individual, especially in cases of emergencies, and with the latter, there was the control by committees, all subject to higher authorities.

****

To be well off, as regards worldly goods, has its disadvantages which eventually may have disastrous and possibly fatal consequences. This in spite of the best efforts of those concerned.

The unfortunate example which illustrates this predicament concerned one of my patients. He was an exceptionally clever designer of intricate packaging.

He called me in one day, as he had a pain in his chest when he took a breath. This was associated with a dry cough which aggravated the pain.

He had a normal temperature, but on examination, movement of the left side of his chest was restricted when he took a breath. I felt that he should be investigated in hospital, and advised that he be admitted by ambulance to avoid undue exertion. I could not make a definite diagnosis but there was an aura of impending collapse. He shrugged my fears off as absurd, saying he would drive to London and consult his Harley Street doctor. He decided to call at his office first to let them know where he would be if he was wanted.

Feeling better, he attempted to run up the stairs of his office, when he collapsed.

A blister on his left lung, from an old injury, had burst.

His Harley Street doctor was sent for, who, after examination, decided he could go home by ambulance, and he would follow. My patient's wife telephoned me and asked me to be present when the other doctor visited.

This I did, and was duly introduced to the Harley Street personality. The physician from Harley Street looked at me. Then he turned to the patient and said,

"I had no idea that you had a village doctor!"

He had brought a pathologist from King's College Hospital with him. This remark brought a rejoinder from the pathologist:- "Dr. Robinson is a colleague at King's from the Ear, Nose, and Throat Department."

After further investigations, the patient was advised rest, and later made a good recovery.

Some months later, I was asked to visit the patient again, as he had

had some vomiting associated with abdominal pain. When I examined him, I diagnosed acute appendicitis, and, in my opinion, the appendix threatened to perforate with subsequent peritonitis. I advised immediate admission to hospital and operation.

Again he demurred, rang up his Harley Street doctor, who had him admitted to the London Clinic.

In the meantime, the appendix had ruptured, and so the vital symptoms had disappeared. Unfortunately, the perforation was in a peritoneal pocket in the pelvis and led to a localised infection. My notes had not been sent to the clinic. Of course, general peritonitis would have been unmistakable.

After weeks of investigation by various specialists, he suddenly had an abscess rupture through the posterior wall of his pelvis, when his condition rapidly deteriorated, and in spite of the best professional help at the clinic, he died.

He was nursed by one of Rennie's old colleagues from King's, who when she visited us, told us she had had a long talk with the widow.

Rennie's one time colleague described how the specialists at the clinic had done everything they could to save him, but in vain.

What a tragedy.

One of my patients was a hypochondriac, who enjoyed describing the 'agonies' from which she suffered. Her main anxiety was the fear that the 'agonies' would either combine with horrendous results, or even worse try to destroy each other, which might produce an even worse, cataclysm.

When she entered the surgery, if it so happened that there was an interlude at the time, I enjoyed hearing about these mythical agonies. More often, during a busy time, my heart would sink, for she would wait until the last patient except for herself had gone, then enter with a beaming smile to relate the latest efforts of the 'agonies' to disconcert her. On such occasions I sometimes felt that the 'agonies' disconcerted me far more!

There she would sit, with a seraphic smile, gesticulating with her plump arms and hands to reinforce her description of the 'agonies' she was conjuring up, whilst she talked and talked. They were little but fierce 'agonies' running up and down her arms or legs. Sometimes they were in her chest or tummy, chasing each other around. After pouring out these remarkable symptoms. She would ask, with a beaming smile:-

"Is it serious, Doctor?"

One day she surpassed herself. This time it was not the 'agonies', it was a far more serious possible eventuality.

"Doctor," she asked, "If the gasses of the heart and the gasses of the stomach were to meet, whatever would happen?"

"Do you smoke?" I enquired gravely.

"No," she replied.

Then I assured her, "You have nothing to fear."

Then suddenly her expression lightened, and she started to laugh so wholeheartedly, that perforce I, too, had to join in!

One day on a visit to a new patient in Bexley, I glanced out of the window, and saw what looked like a fleet of hot-air balloons. They were stationary and appeared to be tethered. Curiosity made me look again and I realised that they were canopies tethered around trees and shrubs.

My patient explained that he was a butterfly farmer. Of course I realised then, that I had seen him on television. He was the Mr. Newman who entertained so many of us. He had a large professional connection and sent specimens all over the world. The breeding of silkworms enthralled me. To see the very fine strands of silk being wound off the cocoons, and then to watch a number of strands being spun together to form threads of silk was most impressive.

Even all those years ago, he was breeding endangered species. His work and devotion to it must have comprised one of the pioneer efforts to protect and save numerous species.

The practice continued to increase and I hoped, in a year or two, to have reached the magic income of just over two thousand pounds a year. This was the borderline, which once crossed, would enable me to have a partner. This, as my hospital attendances were increasing, would soon be essential. Our son, Waring, was about two years of age when he complained of earache and speedily developed signs of mastoiditis.

After the tragic death of our nephew, we were naturally anxious to do all we could by getting the best advice. I got our child admitted to the Children's Hospital, at Sydenham, and asked my chief, Mr. Hope, Ear, Nose, and Throat surgeon at King's College Hospital, to see him.

Unfortunately, at the time, he was at his consulting rooms in the

West End of London, and found his journey to Sydenham through London very difficult, as many roads were closed and others diverted for the Royal Jubilee celebrations. When at last be arrived, he examined Waring and operated forthwith. The operation was not a simple one, and it was with relief that Mr. Hope assured Rennie and me that our son would soon be able to leave hospital and come home.

Waring was devoted to his mother, and his distress at even such a short break away from her was piteous.

Fortunately nowadays, with the protection of antibiotics, mothers can stay in hospital with young children, and thus on the part of the small patients avoid the desolate feeling of rejection.

Personal experience of such heart-rending anxiety has helped me to understand and sympathise with other parents.

Another day, at out-patients at the Children's Hospital in Sydenham, a young mother brought her daughter, aged about four, with a letter from her doctor. She suffered from nasal obstruction and frequent feverish colds.

The child had a very anti-doctor expression on her face and her lips were tightly closed. As the nurse lifted her onto the examination chair, I read the doctor's letter.

"Open your mouth so that I can peep inside," I said.

At that the mother exclaimed,

"T'aint no use Doctor. We had an awful time at the surgery. Wild horses wouldn't make her open her mouth!"

I looked at the very determined little patient and remarked:-

"Wild horses, how wonderful. Have you ever seen a real wild horse?" She shook her head. I realised I had her attention. "I can tell you a tale about a wild horse mother and her little baby boy wild horse." I began:-

"The mother wild horse was very worried because her baby wild horse couldn't close his mouth. He couldn't eat or drink and was getting weak.

So the wild horse mother took him to see a 'vet', that was a wild horse doctor.

The 'vet' looked into the baby's mouth which was wide open and what do you think he saw?

He saw a blue ball stuck between the teeth of the baby wild horse at the back of his mouth."

By this time the child was listening wide-eyed. I went on:-

"The horse doctor put a towel over the teeth of the baby horse and gently pulled the blue ball out of the little wild horse's mouth.

The baby horse was so glad to be able to shut his mouth again that he went frisking and galloping all over the place."

I saw that my patient's mouth had opened wide.

"Let me just peep inside there and I will tell you what I see," I coaxed.

I had no difficulty and was able to reply to the doctor, that if there was no improvement before she was seven, removal of her tonsils and adenoids would be advisable.

I handed the letter to the mother, the little girl jumped down and threw her arms round me and kissed me. That was an unexpected surprise award and one I have never forgotten. It might appear to some that such an approach would take up too much time during a busy session. Yet, having detached the child's attention away from the ordeal that she was dreading, the few minutes lost were well worthwhile.

I hope that the mother learnt from the incident. Certainly at the time she was relieved that there had been no difficulty.

That day, I returned home to find Rennie was far from well. She had exhausted even her seemingly boundless energy, and was so debilitated that she had a recurrence of an ailment which she developed during her childhood, following the death of her mother. She was examined thoroughly for sensitivity to various foods.

Animal fats were the cause of severe attacks of migraine with blinding headaches, associated with vomiting and prostration. Blood examination revealed a marked degree of anaemia. It was months before she regained her full strength, which thankfully, she did.

Waring was now old enough to start school, which meant all three children were at school.

Unfortunately, the private infants school Waring was attending, and at which he was happy, had to close when the proprietress retired. This was reminiscent of my own kinder-garden days but in his case was not associated with any black marks. His next school was a Crusaders' School in Sidcup. Soon afterwards, he started talking out of the side of his mouth. This habit proved very difficult to correct, and Rennie and I both wondered why he should have developed such a peculiar idiosyncrasy. Waring was keen on the school sports and on sports day we found his favourite master 'talking out of the side of his mouth'! He was an excellent teacher and a favourite with all the boys.

The years were passing and the international situation was increasingly grave.

The 'gay twenties' were now past, and the third decade of the twentieth century was entering its last two years. We offered to take one of the Jewish refugees fleeing Hitler's atrocious persecution. As already described, the offer was accepted, and she was the only one of her family to survive.

The practice had at last increased sufficiently to attract a partner and I sought the help of the British Medical Association in 1938.

During the Spring of that year Rennie told me she was expecting our fourth baby. The probable date would be in October.

Meanwhile the British Medical Association had sent all its members a questionnaire in view of the possibility of war. This form asked for qualifications, age, experience, would you volunteer?

I was very conscious of the underserved stigma of 'dodging the column' during World War I. At my age, a married man with three children and another expected, I would not volunteer, but agreed to abide by the decision of the Association's Committee. Meanwhile various applicants for the partnership came for an interview. Among them some doctors with better qualifications than I had! One of them appeared ideal but insisted on an equal share. At first I felt that I should have a major share as the practice had been to a large extent my creation, but it was pointed out that I would of course be the senior partner. Pride soon mollified, I readily agreed and instructions for drawing up the agreement went ahead.

Meanwhile practice routine continued, and one summer day when the school holidays had just ended and surgery attendances were at the seasonal minimum, a schoolgirl whom I had been treating for a debilitating illness was my last patient that morning. I had recently treated her for what is now recognised as glandular fever. The family had just returned from their seaside holiday.

"Doctor," she pleaded, "don't let my parents know that I have come to see you, as it would worry them."

"So long as it isn't anything serious, which they should know about, I won't mention it" I promised.

"I want to do well this term," she continued, " but I feel so lacking in energy, that I decided to pluck up my courage and ask you to put a little life into me."

This request, made with such innocence was particularly appealing. I replied that it was customary for the recent illness she suffered from to be followed by a long period of lassitude before the patient regained full vigour.

I pointed out some weeks had already passed since her attack and, although she did not realise it, she was already on the brink of a full recovery.

To encourage her I prescribed a tonic and assured her, that when school restarted, she would feel her strength and confidence returning.

I wrote out a prescription for a tonic and told her to collect the bottle from the chemist that afternoon.

After she had left, and as she was the last patient that morning, I took all the prescriptions over to the chemist, who now dispensed for panel patients and private ones as well. We always discussed each prescription to avoid any error, and generally had a short friendly chat. On this occasion, I mentioned the young girl's request that as she felt so weak would I put a little life into her? This turned out to be a mistake on my part as I discovered next Saturday morning.

It was a lovely summer day and the High Street was full of shoppers as I walked along it. Suddenly I was hailed by the chemist's wife from across the road:-

"Doctor, what is this I hear? That you have put a little life into one of your lady patients?"

There was an almost audible gasp from pedestrians on both sides of the road.

I was aghast, and wished myself anywhere other than the High Street. There was a silence as those present awaited my reply. I was so taken aback that it took me a while to formulate an answer. At last I said:

"It is true, I was asked to do as you say but I wrote out a prescription and referred her to your husband."

Thus unwittingly making matters worse.

Who or what was to blame for this contretemps?

The innocence of the young schoolgirl? My folly in telling the tale to the chemist? His in telling his wife, or her questioning of me across a busy street?

Whatever the answer, another patient had no solution to all her problems. She was a charge-nurse at Bexley Mental Hospital and came to me to discuss her troubles. Her husband was a charge-nurse on the male side and the family lived outside the hospital, which explains how they came to be my patients. The wife appeared to be in good physical health but was suffering from the onset of the menopause, with feelings of depression and anxiety.

In spite of her professional calling I soon realised that she had delusions. Our house now had the surgery attached and I held morning and evening sessions. This patient suddenly stopped addressing me as doctor and called me 'Sir' instead. One morning, when she had been trying to get some relief from her anxieties, after trying to comfort her, I had prescribed a placebo rather than a sedative.

"Thank you Sir, but I shall have to wait until tomorrow to call at the chemist," she remarked.

"Why wait till tomorrow?" I asked. "The chemist is on your way home."

"That wouldn't be right," she said. "I must keep to the right. If I went to the left, Satan would catch me. He's always following me." Like a flash my mind went back to those terrible nightmares of my childhood when 'Satan' chased me with his trident. I managed to allay this immediate anxiety by giving her some tablets for the day. She turned to me and said

"I know who you are, Sir, you are St. John, the Baptist, and that's why you live here opposite the church of St. John's!"

By now I was completely out of my depth, so I offered to run her home as she was trembling with apprehension. She refused the offer and set off to the right, having to circumvent the centre of the town.

What should I do?

I decided to tell her husband as I felt he should know, otherwise a tragedy might occur. This I did in strict confidence. Alas, I never saw either of them again.

So far, I have shown what an astonishing variety of human activities are to be found in a small town. Soon after I had qualified and before I met Rennie, a representative called to see me and showed me examples of beautiful mezzotint engravings in colour. They were of paintings by Turner, Corot, Constable and other famous artists. I may have only a four colour vision, but these lovely pictures fascinated me.

Rennie was delighted with them and they have given us great

pleasure over the years.

One day I was asked to see a patient at home, not that he was unable to come to the surgery, but he was unavoidably detained at home. Please would I help the caller, his rather distracted wife? I fixed an approximate time and called a little too early. His wife was apologetic and said

"Doctor, my husband is an engraver of mezzotints and is taking a print. He won't be long. He has a bad pain in his back, which is interfering with his work."

I immediately hoped that I could see the Master at work and explained how I came to be so interested.

I was taken down to his workroom. There was a large table similar to a billiard one, and the engraver was just removing his last print of a limited edition.

His wife introduced me and he asked to be excused for a moment whilst he examined this final print. Satisfied, he took a scriber and scored a huge X over the plate. The end of a limited edition.

To me it seemed sacrilege but, of course, necessary.

He then told me of the difficulty he had with his engraving owing to the pain in his back. I examined him in bed and found a very tender spot in the musculature of his backbone. This I injected with a local anaesthetic which gave immediate relief. He was delighted, and began to describe the art of mezzotint engraving. To my surprise, among other details, I learned that the final etching had all the colours applied to the plate before a print was taken.

There was a garden party in the late summer, I forget for what charity or local purpose, but there was a fortune teller there who was a genuine Romany. She had a great reputation as a soothsayer. I had always tended to scoff at the awe with which palmistry or fortune telling was regarded. This time Rennie and I thought that we would have our fortunes told just for fun and to support the cause.

Rennie entered the 'sanctum' first and was surprised at what the gypsy soothsayer told her. Two points were certainly plausible. One was she would never be rich, and the other that she would never be the last on a bus! How very true. First and foremost in any venture, always with an anticipation of excitement shining in her eyes, was typical of my wife.

Next came my turn, she asked to see my palms. I held them out before her, she took one look and said with a note of surprise,

"You see with your fingers, they ask questions and seek the answers, which you try to find."

This struck me as unusually perceptive. She went on,

"What do you do with those sensitive fingers? They are not associated with music but they tell you things, that you otherwise cannot make out.

I think you must be a veterinary surgeon. Your patients cannot tell you their symptoms"

How near she was. Of course most of my work was with young children.

She also said I had a long life ahead of me, but that was only a possibility.

Since this experience, I feel that these soothsayers, at any rate the best of them, possess an extensive store of knowledge of human behaviour, attainments and eccentricities.

This is another form of the lore handed done from ages past and on a par with the knowledge of medicinal herbs and water divining. A heritage from our forebears to be treasured.

1938, the year of 'Peace in our time'. A period of bogus tranquillity. 'Who threw dust in the eyes of whom?' All of us have seen the picture of Neville Chamberlain alighting from the aircraft flourishing the famous or infamous piece of paper.

History, it is to be hoped, will reveal the truth. Those priceless months, that were the final gestation period of World War Two, gained a vital respite for this country with a chance to rearm and build an airforce which saved democracy from doom in 1940.

Christmas 1938 was the last before the storm broke.

We all still hoped that peace would be preserved.

At St. Laurence we had a memorable family party. Father Christmas arrived, with a sledge drawn by a cardboard reindeer with a shining eye which blinked, as it nodded its head, when Father Christmas found a present for each child and adult. Rennie was in her element and kept alive the joy of Christmas with its message of love and goodwill.

The fateful New Year, 1939, inevitably soon followed the brief rejoicing of Christmastide.

A brief resume of the international events of the previous five years reveals the insidious spread of international aggression.

1935:

Mao's Communists march 1000 miles into China. Chiang fighting on two fronts against Mao and the Japanese.

1936:

Civil war in Spain. Abdication of Edward VIII. Italian troops occupy Abyssinnia.

1937:

Palestine. British plan Arab and Jewish separate states. The Japanese capture Nanking.

1938:

Whittle builds first jet engine. Anschluss between Germany and Austria. Anti-Jewish outbreaks in Nazi Germany.

1939:

Franco takes Barcelona and creates fascist Spain.

Czechoslovakia absorbed by Nazi Germany.

France called up reservists.

Almost incredible non-aggression pact between Hitler and Stalin.

Third September Britain declared war on Germany, following German invasion of Poland.

Civilian life at the start of the New Year on the surface continued normally, but with a haunting fear of war.

The Government acted speedily to make the most of the treasured interval of breathing space. First and foremost were the air defences: The invention of 'Radar' with its early warning screen and the vast energy throughout the country poured into production of Spitfire, and Hurricane fighter aircraft.

It seemed that almost overnight additional precautions were taken, with the creation of numerous air-raid shelters and an army of air-raid wardens and of course the Home Guard. The fear was that, if war started, the Germans would use poison gas. When an easterly wind was blowing, ships could discharge a huge blanket of poison gas which would envelop London and vast tracts of the country. Gas masks were provided in huge numbers and even special infant protective suits. These were terrifying for the babies and fortunately were never required. Every adult and each schoolchild was provided with a mask to carry with them to work or to school.

My future practice partner was in the reserve and was soon called up for service in the R.A.M.C., and so the proposed partnership had to be abandoned, at any rate for the time being. Our fourth child, a boy, was born on the twenty-eighth of March. From his birth, he was a happy and contented child and started to smile at an incredibly early age. His sister, Paddy, claimed him as her special charge, as her elder sister had looked upon Waring as hers! He was christened Geoffrey Morris Waring, and Morris, (an old family name) has been universally used.

One day I had had a long operating session at the children's hospital. When I had finished and seen the patients in the wards, and as was customary, had a cup of tea with the anaesthetist and resident, I anticipated a speedy return home, and a short rest before evening surgery.

As I reached the entrance hall, and looked at the notice board to change 'In' to 'Out' against my name, I saw it had already been altered to 'Out'. At that moment the porter said

"I thought you had left, Sir."

"Oh no" I replied, "there was a long list this afternoon."

He then said,

"Well your car has gone, and I thought the driver was you, for he waved goodbye, Sir."

To my dismay, the Humber Snipe had been stolen.

Apart from feeling marooned at the hospital, I had other duties at Bexley, including evening surgery and some visits. All I could do was inform the police, the insurance company, and then start for home by bus and train.

The following morning, I heard from the police that my car had been found with the engine racing, and boiling furiously. I was asked to collect it. Fortunately the constable who had found the car had switched off the engine.

We had a second car, which was my wife's, and she used it to take the children to school and for shopping. We drove to where the Humber Snipe had been left, and after some discussion with the police, we drove both the cars home.

The next morning after breakfast, I went out to start the Humber Snipe. As I pressed the starter, the engine fired and then came a horrible tearing sound and the engine seemed to fly to pieces.

I could see, as soon as I lifted the bonnet, that the sump was fractured, and a connecting rod was sticking out of the gaping gash. Such a calamity could hardly have happened at a more critical time. The war clouds were threatening to break any day. Indeed I had already approached the Building Society about the mortgage, in the event of hostilities.

The car was towed away for an estimate. The insurance company having been informed, I asked the garage to await the insurance company's engineer before they did anything.

The garage reported that the engine was beyond repair and should be replaced by a new one.

"Wait until the insurance engineer has been and made out his report," I repeated again.

The manager of the garage grinned and replied:

"A new engine is being supplied. We have already ordered one."

"On no account fit it until the insurance company has agreed," I instructed. In spite of my order, however, the garage staff went ahead and installed the new engine. The insurance engineer examined the old engine and reported that the big end had been fitted with a split pin which was too small, this caused the failure of the big end, and the company refused all liability. I applied to the R.A.C. who sent down their inspector and he agreed with the engineer's report. Almost simultaneously, war was declared, and any hope of my paying that bill faded. The garage retained the car as security, when I was called up for service.

But for the threat of hostilities, I think an offer of part payment for the new engine would have been made.

The B.M.A. secretary wrote to tell me that the committee decided in view of my past service in the Territorials that my name should be forwarded to the War Office for consideration for service in the R.A.M.C.

This was August and I was anxious to safeguard our house as far as possible. This meant having an air raid shelter for the family in the basement and an efficient 'blackout'.

I heard from my friend, Gerald Rudolf, that he had been called up and had been appointed to the First General Hospital R.A.M.C. with the rank of captain.

In view of the expected air raids and poison gas attacks, he and his wife, Rosemary, suggested that our two families shared their home in Clevedon, Somerset. We accepted this offer gladly. Meanwhile I heard from the War Office that with my specialist qualifications, I would be offered a temporary commission as Major in due course. In the meantime would I be prepared to serve as a unit medical officer in the B.E.F, on a temporary basis?

Still allergic to the slur of 'dodging the column' I foolishly agreed, thereby landing myself in severe financial difficulties. I should have refused to serve as a unit medical officer. War was declared on the third of September, and on the ninth I was called up as a unit medical officer and told to report forthwith to the Second General Hospital R.A.M.C. in the Aldersot area.

Somehow we managed. My wife and the children and I had driven down to Clevedon to a warm welcome from Rosemary.

The two other G.P.s in Bexley offered to look after my Bexley practice whilst I was serving in the R.A.M.C.

Things happened so speedily then, that some details are blurred.

Greatly relieved, knowing Rennie and the children were in Somerset with Rosemary, I reported to the 2nd General Hospital. When I arrived, there was a practice emergency alert of a gas attack, and the whole area was deserted except for some personnel wearing gas masks. Eventually the all clear went and I saw the Second-in-Command, who told me to take a few days leave to obtain my uniform, and be prepared to report at any time, as the hospital was under orders for overseas. I did have more than a day or two, but a tailor in Bristol rapidly measured me, and had my uniform ready in forty eight hours!

There was a hurried goodbye before I joined the hospital, to find that it was already about to depart for France. I had packed all my specialist paraphernalia in a compact case and, in my hurry, found that I had left it behind. I managed to telephone Rennie, and she rushed to Temple Meads station and told the station-master that the case must reach me before the hospital left. To my relief it arrived just in time. What a difference there was embarking compared with the First World War. Instead of the cheers and flag waving, there was a grim sad farewell from onlookers.

We disembarked at Cherbourg and there was time to stroll down to the town and try out my French.

My tutor had been adamant on pronunciation, and had persevered until my brother, Oliver, and I came up to his exacting standard.

At this early stage of the war all British personnel were greeted with boisterous rapture. It was a beautiful September day, and a market was in full swing on the quayside. The whole area exuded bonhomie, and my first impression of the French was far from warlike. When I opened my mouth, my pronunciation conveyed the impression that I was conversationally fluent. Quite the opposite, and it was some time before I could calm down the torrent of welcome. At last I escaped from the greetings of stallholders, and as I left I could still hear the chattering at the market, mingled with "O, la, las" and the laughter of children.

I rejoined my Unit at the station where all was hustle and sorting out.

By this time all ranks were hungry and longing for refreshment. The quartermaster shouted, "You will all have a meal on the train, don't worry." This did not deter one bright, (or not so bright), individual, who made tea in a large dish with boiling water from the locomotive. This had varying effects on those who sampled it. There was a subtle but pervasive element of sulphurated hydrogen about it.

This Satanic aroma did not appeal to me.

The train started for our unknown destination, shrewdly expected to be Dieppe, as proved to be a correct guess. To my surprise, General Hospitals 1 and 2 were side by side.

To my pleasure, there was Gerald Rudolf to greet me!

Apart from this surprise, there were no outstanding events during this period. In fact it was the start of the phoney war. The lovely weather continued for a week or two and all personnel were able to make the most of it.

Patients were few, and those treated were the result of accidents or minor complaints.

As the B.E.F. settled down medical officers were detailed to various units. For some time I stayed at the hospital. We lived in tents, and the easy life we led prompted me to do what I could to make my tent as comfortable as possible. So I made a bed, a table, and some other items.

The second-in-command came to see me, and when he saw my attempts at furnishings, he exclaimed

"It's like a prostitute's boudoir!"

Roars and roars of laughter followed this sally. This easy existence soon ended, when I was posted as unit M.O. to the petrol park 2nd Corps.

I was given a railway warrant and set off with another officer for the same region. We got on well and it was with regret, that we found when we arrived at our destination, that our postings were in different areas. As we parted he said how much he had enjoyed meeting me, especially as it had been something he had rather dreaded. He had feared that, as I was a teetotaller, I would be very 'pi' and a likely 'Godbotherer'. What a description! How easy it is to jump to wrong conclusions.

I met the C.O. and members of the mess and felt more 'at home'.

****

The weather changed, it became colder and wet. The winter of 1939/1940 was to be one of the most severe for years. Just as I had established a routine, I was posted to the Ammunition Park 2nd. Corps. This was a larger unit, and to my surprise one of my old Bexley patients was the C.O. This was an unexpected reunion and brought back memories of Bexley to both of us. My area now was much larger as it included my previous unit the Petrol Park.

There were three non-combatant officers - the Padre, a Scot, the Liaison officer, Monsieur Le Bat and I. Our respective jobs brought us together a lot. If not another 'Three Musketeers'. we tried to help as a triumvirate. The Padre looked after the 'souls', the Liaison Officer harmonised relations with the French, and I tagged along, as a curer of bodily ills. Whilst I was having a comparatively easy time and enjoying seeing so much of the country and its inhabitants, my wife was enduring what can only be described as hardship. Rennie not only looked after our four children, her three nieces, and Rosemary's son, Noel, (while both Rennie's sister and Rosemary were away) but in addition she had several evacuees from London and Bristol. She laboured from morning till night. One day a young woman called to see her, and after hearing about all the tasks which Rennie had to squeeze into the twenty-four hours, she sweetly enquired

"But can't you do something for the war effort?"

Rennie's reply was short and to the point, she was doing more than sitting on her backside, asking damn fool questions!

In wartime, life on the home front is very different from that in the field. At home it is one long and tedious struggle against almost intolerable conditions and shortages, to which there seems no end, whilst in the forces it varies from months of boredom to sudden explosions of frenzied activity.

During this period of calm in France I was reported to headquarters as a potential spy.

Having considerable leisure I decided to take up sketching. As long as I confined my activities to indoors, all was well, but I had seen, growing near a drainage ditch, a willow tree, perhaps bush is a better word, for it had been having a war of its own with the local farming community.

In spite of murderous onslaughts by cattle and humans, it had managed to endure. When I came across it, I was astonished at the complexity of its vigorous shoots attempting to survive in a maze of twists and turns that would have reduced to simplicity the fabled Gordian Knot of antiquity.

I went out with my stool, sketching pad and pencils. It is difficult to explain why this task should have been so absorbing. I failed to notice first one, and then another, local coming to watch, if I turned round they just disappeared. When I returned to mess, I was told that the C.O. wished to see me. It was then that I learned that a German 'paratrooper', disguised as a British Medical Officer, had been seen behaving suspiciously, making sketches of landmarks.

So ended my out of doors 'artistic' efforts.

Later talking about this with the Padre, I drew his attention to the scene one late afternoon, when it was bathed in a subtle almost Turnerseque evening glow.

He looked, and then said "Aye, Mon, but it canna compare with the Moors of Rannoch!"

We were to hear much more of the 'Moors of Rannoch', in due course.

As November drew on to its final two weeks, an outbreak of coughs and colds made its appearance amongst both the civil population and the B.E.F. The irritating coughs were distressing not only for the infected men, but also because their comrades frequently had their night's sleep interrupted.

When I tried to get supplies of aspirin and cough linctus from our quartermaster's stores, to my astonishment I was met with a blank refusal. The quartermaster's idea was, if news of an epidemic amongst the B.E.F. reached the enemy, the result might be disastrous. It was no use my pointing out that contagions, however mild, had no preference for individual armies, and that the Germans were probably in worse straits, as these epidemics generally spread from the East. I was a sole medico and I did not wish to cause trouble by referring the matter to base.

I had already set up an M.I. (medical inspection) room in a cottage, which had been requisitioned. Only the lower floor had so far been used. There was an upper attic room reached by rickety stairs. If it was large enough, I could use it as a temporary sickbay.

I climbed the stairs and stepped into the past!

The loft was dimly illuminated by light filtering through a dusty fanlight. The first thing I noticed was that the interior of the roof had been covered with sheets of tin. I recognised these tin sheets. They were formed from army four-gallon petrol tins after the petrol had been used. This had been common practice by the B.E.F. in World War I to reduce draughts during the winters, also to stop any rain dripping in. As my vision improved, I saw evidence of a hasty departure. There was a broken penknife, an old 'housewife', several old photographs, which crumbled to dust when touched. Some half consumed cigarettes, numerous burnt out stubs and candle ends stuck on the tops of cigarette tins. There was a billycan, cigarette cards and some old letters. All just shapes, mouldy and decayed almost beyond recognition.

There was no time for dwelling on the past, although I hoped to find out which unit in the First World War had left these so forlorn and sad remnants.

I had the loft cleared, cleaned, and bunks set up for six men. So I had an unofficial advanced dressing station. More serious cases were sent to base hospital.

To ease the irritating coughs, I bought some cornflour and blackcurrant jam. These two made a linctus which, whilst it may not have been pharmaceutically perfect, still helped.

The Padre came to see how the sick were faring. He tasted the linctus, smacked his lips and observed predictably

"Ah mon, but it canna compare with blackcurrants from the Moor of Rannoch."

It was soon December, the epidemic dwindled and finally ended. Letters from home were eagerly awaited, and we all were almost unapproachable, whilst they were read and re-read. To add to our hopes, there were rumours of leave for Christmas. I found out that my leave would not be until late January at the earliest. I wondered how on earth I could manage to arrange sending Christmas presents. After some thought, I wrote to Gamages enclosing a cheque and a list of names with sex and ages where necessary. I included funny tie-on labels with drawings of, for instance, 'Mr. Spring of Clockwork House' and other daft ideas. Gamages were very helpful and sent most appropriate gifts, but alas, the Censor removed the labels. Obviously I was still under suspicion as a possible enemy 'paratrooper'. I was O.C. mess and I tried to get some change from army diet. When I was in Aubigny, I was able to get some salmon for the mess just before Christmas. This was certainly a change and went down well. Even the Padre approved, but he could not help himself from smacking his lips and coming out with the old refrain, "Ah, Mon, that was guid but it canna compare with the salmon from the loch by the Moor of Rannoch."

Christmas came and went and thoughts were all on leave. Mine would not be until early spring.

I was asked by the local doctor, if I could help him sometimes. When official duties permitted, I was only too pleased to do so. My first patients were two sisters. They were very depressed after the recent epidemic.

They lived together in a semi-detached house with a bay front window. In the centre of the bay was the stuffed body of a black and tan terrier in an attitude of expectant devotion. The sisters had both lost their men during the First World War. The elder was a widow and the younger was to have been married as soon as her fiancé returned on leave.

Before war broke out in 1914, the two couples had enjoyed such happy times together, and the terrier had been their constant companion.

After the war the sisters cared for the little dog with fond memories of past happy occasions. When the terrier died of old age, they had the body stuffed.

There were tears in their eyes as they told me this tale, which revived thoughts of what might have been.

Touching as the story was, it seemed a bit macabre to me. However, they were charming and interested when they heard that I was Mess Officer, and they introduced me to a bee-keeper. He was an Anglophile, and when he heard that I was mess officer he insisted on providing the mess with some of his best honey. I told the members of the mess the poignant tale of the two sisters and the stuffed dog. The mess were pleased to send their appreciation and thanks for the delicious honey to the bee-keeper. I was of course delighted to convey this message to our French friends. The Padre agreed with all this, nevertheless, could not refrain from adding the inevitable,

"Ah, Mon, but it cannot compare with the heather boney from the Moor of Rannoch."

By this time I felt that I had heard more than enough of the marvels of the Moor of Rannoch, but held my tongue.

Frosts were severe and falls of snow soon added to road hazards. Only approved drivers were allowed to drive and our triumvirate soon had a driver from the petrol park. He was a graded 'fitter' but a worse driver I had never met. Of course the roads were treacherous, but his driving was too dangerous to continue. So I ordered him out and took over the wheel myself.

On our return I enquired as to the fitness of the official driver. I was told that a 'fitter' was a mechanical engineer and a recognised driver.

I asked to see him again and when he appeared looking terrified, I asked him how on earth, if he was a qualified mechanic, could he drive so abominably?

His reply was,

"When I joined up I was asked my trade, and I told them I was a qualified 'fitter', I'm actually a gents' outfitter."

He had been too scared to tell anyone, and as he was useless on the mechanical side, he had been posted as driver for the M.O. I do not know what eventually happened to him, but certainly the army could do with a 'gents' outfitter'. In future I drove myself, often the roads were pitted with ice and then suddenly became like an ice-rink. Driving became hazardous, and to get a grip on the icy surfaces, I bandaged the wheels, when no grit was available.

One day I had the opportunity to add a change to the diet.

I had seen and ordered a selection of French cheeses. They were soft Camembert cheeses and at their best 'ripeness'.

The Padre cut into his cheese and exclaimed in alarm,

"Ah, but it stinks!"

I replied,

"Ah, Mon but it cannot compare with the...."

I got no further for roars of laughter.

We heard no more of the 'Moor of Rannoch' at least for a long time, and I felt a degree of self reproach for causing him some undeserved embarrassment.

The winter months were finally over and my leave came in late

April. The phoney war was nearing its end, but the B.E.F. was still living a placid existence, and wondering if the war would become a semi-permanent war of attrition.

Seven days leave seemed almost unbelievable, yet the day came and I left France in great spirits. The channel crossing was uneventful, and I soon caught the train for Bristol's Templemead station. On arriving there I had two changes to make and time was getting on. The first change for Yatton went smoothly, as that train was waiting for the arrival of the London express. At Yatton I heard that the last train for Clevedon had left. The next would be at 6 a.m. in the morning and I had the frustrating experience of seeing the precious hours of daylight disappearing, as I wondered whatever should I do. The train returned from Clevedon, and would be prepared for the morning's early departure. I was faced with the prospect of waiting all night, as I watched the few passengers alight.

****

Then the engine driver stepped out of the cab to be hailed by the station master, who told him of my plight. He came over and said to me "We will run a 'special' to get you home." This he did, and I was the only passenger, with a whole train to myself! My gratitude was inexpressible and the driver refused any compensation for his loss of time.

Carrying my bag and walking briskly, I felt tired but both elated and joyfully expectant as I reached home.

It was quite late and the children were asleep in bed. Poor Rennie, who had just recovered from an attack of laryngitis, was also fast asleep. She had gone to bed, when I was not on the last train that day. As soon as she heard me ring, she rushed downstairs to greet me, but could only speak in a faint hoarse whisper, the legacy of the laryngitis.

We both treasure the memory of that reunion as we enjoyed an exciting midnight feast. I told her of the kindness of the engine driver running a 'special', and after further exchange of news, tired out, we went to bed.

We were awakened by our youngest, now about a year and a half old, who each morning would jump into his mother's bed for a cuddle. On this occasion, he shouted in dismay,

"Mummy. Who is that man in bed with you?"

When he discovered the man was his father, all was well and we were a happy trio.

I cannot remember doing anything special during that seven days, to be a united family again was all that mattered. The time passed all too quickly and before we realised it, I had to return to France.

The situation in Calais was tense. I knew my brother, Oliver, was there but there was no chance of getting in touch with him. My brief view of the town was confined to the station. I saw that a condition of remarkably orderly turmoil existed. Time was obviously of the utmost importance, and almost before I realised what was happening I was in the train speeding out of the town. Arrived at my unit's H.Q., I was told that the 2nd Corps was about to move up into Belgium.

Everyone was expecting the order at any moment. I had difficulty in preparing to organise the medical side at such short notice. By the next morning the unit was fully prepared including my small section. We waited all day, and still no order. Of course we were the equivalent of the baggage trains of the armies of old. About midday a dispatch rider skidded to a halt at H.Q., although orders were expected by telephone, the wearied and exhausted state of the rider raised our hopes that his dispatch contained the anticipated order to advance. The adjutant opened the fatal envelope and handed the message to the C.O., who read aloud its contents:

Please inform by return whether your men prefer tinned kippers or tinned pilchards?

To many such a happening, at such a vital time may seem incredible, but it actually occurred. Within a few minutes the order to advance into Belgium arrived in a more official way. We crossed the border, and moved towards Brussels.

Cheering, but now tired, children threw faded flowers of welcome. Though tired as well, the troops received their offerings with waves and smiles. It was no more than a few hours after arriving at Herselles, a surburb of Brussels, and a small town in itself, when air raid warnings started.

So much happened in such a short time that I have only a vague recollection as to where I slept, or where H.Q. was in that small town. A nearby convent opened its doors for casualties, and I started to prepare a dressing station. I was surprised to find the nuns and the Mother Superior such practical people, there was no 'holier than thou art' attitude on their part.

I now learnt that my train from Calais had been the last to get through, German panzers had cut the line.

Near the convent was a chateau, the residence of a Count and Countess. They had been advised to leave at once, and they asked me for my advice. I, of course, knew no more than they did, but with the air raid alarm going full blast, I told them I thought they should take the warning seriously and leave. This they did. Since then, I have often wondered how they got on. Standing near the chateau after they had gone, I heard a sudden crunching of trees, and a plane crashed almost into the side of the building. It was a Spitfire and I could see the young pilot with his slim fingers resting on the joystick.

Recollection of this one casualty is impressed for ever on my memory. It seemed that three happenings were almost simultaneous. The youthful figure in the cockpit. I rushed to try to free him, but my orderly and a sergeant pulled me away, as flames appeared. Then there was the roar of another plane, a Messerschmitt I believe, it wobbled just overhead. I thought it was in trouble, but it was a 'Victory Roll'.

Finally I saw those fingers of youth begin to crinkle in the heat, and I wept.

Later, I learnt that nearby was an R.A.F. airfield and that German fighters patrolled high above waiting for our airmen to return for more ammunition and fuel. Subsequently they were instructed never to exhaust their ammunition before returning to base.

That afternoon I was asked if I would like to see the bodies of refugees, horses, and shot up vehicles, which had been blocking the main roads. I asked if there was any hope that some were only wounded. No, I was told, all wounded had already been taken to hospital, and all corpses, and wrecked vehicles had been unceremoniously tipped off the carriageway to free the road. I declined, I had seen enough for one day.

There followed days and days of marching, without, it seemed to me, any ultimate purpose.

Suddenly, we returned to France and entered Arras, an almost deserted town. We had crossed one of the main German supply routes. We had the ammunition and petrol supplies for the 2nd corps, particularly for our tank squadrons.

At the time I had no idea of the purpose of these apparently almost aimless moves, until I read years later about their strategic and tactical importance.

Our unit formed part of a counter-attack which, if successful, would have changed the whole course of history.

The heads, Lord Gort, Allen Brook and the French Commander in Chief, with their staffs, had met after the fall of the 'impregnable' fort at the Belgian border which formed part of the Maginot line. This fort, invincible by land, was helpless when German paratroopers landed on the roof. They created havoc among the defenders by dropping mortar bombs down the ventilator shafts, followed by the blasting of flame throwers. The German Panzer divisions then broke through and were heading for the Channel ports. The Chiefs of staffs of the Allies decided on a counter-attack. The B.E.F. was to play its part by crossing the German supply route, during one of their regular intervals.

The British tank unit would join with the French one, and together would have cut off the advanced German Panzers, which were racing towards the Channel ports.

Communications were in chaos, and the French Commander decided to take the battle order in person. He set off with his staff in their car. The vehicle was spotted by a German plane and bombed, killing all its occupants. No order therefore reached the French in the Maginot line.

The British tanks were confronted by a crack Panzer unit which they defeated, and the German unit withdrew in disarray.

Further Panzer units were reported moving up to cut off and destroy our troops. Withdrawal was essential, and the German supply line was recrossed without detection. The armour went ahead, whilst the ammunition and petrol parks sought camouflage and shelter in the forest bordering the road. All that night, at regular intervals, we could hear the German supply wagons pouring past. Some of our junior officers wanted to mine the road or to block it by felling trees. The C.O. would have none of it, as it would have given away our presence, and deprive the 2nd. corps of vital ammunition and other supplies. We remained there all day, and at nightfall we rejoined the B.E.F. in Belgium. Rumour upon rumour circulated until we heard the definite news that Belgium had surrendered and its army was disbanded. The chaos on the roads was indescribable. They were blocked for miles with abandoned Belgium army vehicles, some having been destroyed.

Utterly exhausted that night I slept in a cellar in the village street. There were lorries filled with land mines just outside, but I slept throughout an air raid. When I woke, to my astonishment, the village street had been bombed, so as to cause the houses to collapse onto the street, thereby blocking it. Mercifully the wagons with the landmines had escaped. The R.E.M.E. engineers arrived, and in an incredibly short time all obstructing vehicles had been removed or tipped over to the side to free the road. This amazing episode is something I have never forgotten.

That day the C.O. sent for me, and announced, as soon as I arrived, "We are lost." This was not as serious as it sounded, but since the collapse of the Belgium army, our communications with

H.Q., had been cut off. He had also sent for the Padre and the Liaison Officer. When they arrived, the C.O. explained the reason for calling us. With Belgium having surrendered, there was a possibility that any Quislings might take advantage of the opportunity to spread alarm, or leak information. The B.E.F. had their H.Q. near La Panne, and he asked us to make our way there quietly and ask for instructions, whether we should stay where we were, or move. No enemy agent would suspect our trio of non-combatants.

The perimeter had now shrunk considerably, and we had only a mile or so to go. The Germans were steadily shelling a cross road, that we had to get over. We managed it easily, as their shells landed at definite intervals, and we arrived at Allen-Brook's H.Q. as he was having a very short break. He greeted us so calmly,

"Padre, Doc, and Monsieur Lebatt, you are just in time for tea. Please sit down and explain why you have come."

He was given our map reference, looked at the map and observed "You are in no man's land there. Tell your C.O. to move at once." He gave another map reference.

We returned as fast as we could, and the unit withdrew speedily to well within the perimeter.

Thinking about this event later, I suddenly realised what a cunning C.O. he was. If we had been shot up, there was every chance one of us at least would have got back!

****

There were three incidents which I feel are worth recording, but I cannot place then in chronological order due to the whirlwind of impending military disasters at the time.

The first happened when our triumvirate still had a car. It was a Ford two-door saloon, seating four. Padre was driving, the Liaison Officer in the passenger seat, and I had two back seats to myself. We were on a main road, when suddenly there was a low-flying German plane which crossed over the road and changed course to turn and overtake us from the rear. The Padre braked and stopped, the front doors flew open, and out the two leapt for shelter at the roadside. I frantically pushed the back of the passenger seat forward to escape, when the Liaison Officer followed his customary habit of slamming the door shut. Back I went with a flop, and by the time I had re-opened the door, got out, and run a few feet, the plane was overhead. A few more paces and I could see the rear gunner, then the road was cut up as if in a hailstorm, whilst bullets whistled past me on both sides. I hardly had time to breathe before the plane had vanished.

However I enjoyed the last laugh for the others were in a manure heap in which I would have certainly joined then but for the closed door.

The second incident was when we were on foot, wearily plodding, and we overtook a private who was sitting by the roadside. He had his pack on his back and it was bulging. His face looked ghastly as he attempted to rise. He groaned and collapsed, as we stopped to help him.

I freed his shoulder straps, and took a deep breath to lift the pack. It was so light that I nearly fell over. It turned out to be crammed with packets of cigarettes. When he had recovered a bit, the soldier told us that he was in the N.A.A.F.I. stores when the order came to evacuate and destroy what could not be removed. The idea of destroying thousands of cigarettes seemed sacrilege to him. He smoked as many as possible, sometimes thirteen at a time, and crammed as many as he could into his pack. He was of course suffering from carbon monoxide poisoning. He looked upon himself as helping the Allied Cause by depriving the enemy of loot!

The third episode was during a forced march; a lance-corporal ran up to the adjutant to ask permission for a few of the men, who were farm workers, to milk some cows, who were in great distress, as they had not been milked for days. Permission was given, provided they returned at the double. Alas, no milk could be saved, but by the time the men rejoined the unit, they were in a breathless and exhausted state.

Another occurrence was when conditions became so bad that all unnecessary equipment had to be destroyed. I had been asked to see a child in an isolated cottage who was screaming with earache. Fortunately, I still had my case of instruments. The child was about five years old, and had an acute ear infection. On examination I found the eardrum was inflamed and bulging. Fortunately so far there was no evidence of mastoid involvement.

After a few drops of a local anaesthetic, I was able to lance the drum, and the ear discharged freely. I left orders for treatment, and warned against using any fluid or lotion. Next morning I hoped to find the child improved, and went to collect my specialist equipment. To my dismay, it had been thrown into the canal in accord with the order about the destruction of unnecessary equipment. I had lost an auriscope, an opthalmoscope, tuning forks, and other fine and delicate instruments. What possible harm could have come from their use by enemy surgeons?. I felt quite disarmed and useless.

To underline my distress, I saw flight upon flight of enemy bombers dropping their deadly loads on Dunkirk.

I had time to visit yesterday's patient and was glad to find her improving. I took the opportunity of leaving my tea making kit there, Primus stove, two small containers of methylated spirit, paraffin, and some tea.

A defensive force had been rapidly formed from our unit and other base troops. They marched off, with small arms ammunition, mortar bombs, and land mines in the few vehicles remaining. All the rest such as heavy lorries and equipment were destroyed The defensive perimeter was now much smaller. Our scratch defenders held the right flank, vacated by the Belgians, and on the left were the French divisions, who fought magnificently. Evacuation of the B.E.F. and French troops was under way as the perimeter shrank. My unit had been disbanded, and we made our separate ways, either to Dunkirk, or to the beaches at La Panne. This was orderly and completely controlled.

The Padre, the Liason Officer, and I were among the beach parties.

The state of the beach with long queues of men standing in the sea up to their waists, waiting to be evacuated by small boats, must be familiar to all from the television programmes. We were in one of the rows and getting more and more soaked. About a mile along the beach towards Dunkirk, I saw a small boat, which looked precariously beached.

There was a dejected looking figure standing by it. I called the Padre's attention to it, and he said he was sure that it was to evacuate the nuns from the nearby convent. I did not believe that, for the evacuation was probably on its last day. It was May the thirtieth, and the perimeter was almost non-existent. I thought, we should at least make sure that it was not for our troops, and I decided to investigate. Both the others refused to move, afraid that our places in the queue would be lost. I was determined to find out however and resolved to go. This I did, and was surprised to find the other two following me, even though they grumbled about what an absurd chance I was taking. After a trudge over the sand, we eventually reached the boat, which was beached and attended by a depressed looking young naval rating, who was greatly relieved to be able to explain his difficulties. He had been detailed by the commander of his parent ship to ferry troops from the beach to the vessel which was anchored offshore. He disclosed that he was a raw recruit, and was at a loss how to relaunch the boat which was at least twenty foot long.

One of the two outboard engines would not start he went on, when he had tried to steer, the boat turned round and beached itself. Fortunately I spotted a dispatch rider nearby, and managed to attract his attention. I told him to go to the queue we had left, and ask about a dozen men to come help launch the boat. He did this, but while waiting, I looked at the defective motor, and decided that without tools it could not be restarted, so I had it detached and placed in the bottom of the boat. I asked the rating to change the position of the functioning motor to as near the centre of the stern, making sure it did not interfere with the rudder.

Also while waiting, I had time to view the scene before my eyes. There were numerous wrecked craft, half sunken near the shore, dead horses, being washed to and fro in the breakers. Innocent animals, what had they done to deserve such a fate? There were no corpses that I could see, other than these. I believe any human bodies had been discreetly removed. Towards Dunkirk were volumes of smoke, and the sound of detonating bombs. There was very little bombing of the beach, and those bombs which did fall buried themselves deep into the sand and were comparatively harmless.

For some time our rations had consisted of water, bully beef, and hardboiled eggs. A nourishing diet, but it soon became monotonous, especially in the warmth of lovely spring weather. We found ourselves day-dreaming of luscious ice-cool fruit salads, and even delicacies from the Moor of Rannoch! At last help arrived with a number of men from the queue.

None seemed to know anything about boats except myself for the little I knew from dingy sailing. So, perforce I had to do what I could. To my amazement they all jumped to my orders! We managed to get the boat partly afloat, then I told two men to get in and when the rest of us pushed, they were to leap forward as the boat floated free on the first breaker, preventing the boat being again beached. Whether right or wrong it worked and soon we had a boatfull of men afloat, and with the one outboard motor working, our naval rating steered thankfully for the parent ship.

What an astonishing vessel it was. It was a huge coastal barge, which carried coal from Newcastle to ports along the East coast. The defective outboard motor was taken aboard and soon repaired, and off our naval rating sped to the rescue once more.

I was barely conscious of what was happening for now that the strains and anxieties of the past few days were over, we three just flopped down and went fast asleep. What eventually woke me up was the delicious fragrance of freshly baked bread. This sensation recalled to me what 'manna' meant for the Israelites. The loaves must have been baked on board for they were still fresh from the oven. As we munched the fragrant crusts, to our surprise the decks were now brimming with troops, both British and French. Not all were so fortunate, some field ambulances, packed with wounded too severely injured to be moved, volunteered to stay and face captivity rather than forsake their patients.

They faced a bitter future as prisoners.

Curiously, now in my old age, I have had the privilege of meeting one of the nursing orderlies, who had volunteered to remain with the wounded. He told me of the hardships that the units had to suffer. Some had to endure forced marches as far as Poland. Attempts were frequently made to indoctrinate them and afterwards they would be asked "Do you love the Führer?"! After repatriation, the past sacrifice of their liberty on behalf of the severely injured was specifically acknowledged by His Majesty, the King, with a letter of thanks and appreciation of their unselfish devotion to the wounded.

On our rescue vessel, it was with relief that we heard the Commander order, "Full ahead." He was a temporary Lt. RN., and seemed so young to me. He told me that he was in church being married, when the order came for him to join in the rescue of the B.E.F. immediately. The ceremony was quickly completed. He seemed so distressed, that apart from expressing my sympathy I quickly changed the subject. I remarked at the slow progress we appeared to he making compared with so many other boats, which were much smaller.

He explained that there was a strong current parallel with the coastline, and that the maximum speed of our craft was less than this, so he had to steer, taking this into account. Looking over the side I was horrified to see what looked like a minefield. "Not to worry," he said amusedly, "the mines are set at a lower depth than our maximum draft."

Yet he appeared so capable and confident, that he created a feeling of optimism among us all.

Our passage was uninterrupted, and any hostile aircraft seeing us, so slowly wallowing on our way, may have thought either that we were already in a hopeless state, or that we would be here for sinking on their next sortie. Numerous other craft were not so fortunate, and it was heartbreaking to see still blazing wrecks just off Dunkirk. Enormous columns of smoke were belching from the oil storage tanks there, which had been deliberately destroyed by the Allies.

A hospital ship was close inshore and she appeared to us to be in a perilous area of minefields. Later we realised that this was probably the hospital ship which we heard had been sunk. Double summer time was in force, I believe at the end of May, which accounts for our arrival at Ramsgate Harbour at eventide, after what seemed hours and hours of tortoise-like progress. It seemed a miraculous deliverance.

We were all hustled off the vessel almost before we could collect our wits. I had no time to say thank you and express the admiration of all the rescued for what was undoubtedly superb courage and seamanship on the part of our skipper. Unfortunately I cannot recall his name or that of the craft. I fear he had to face at least one more hazardous attempt at succouring the last remnants of our troops from the beech at La Panne. One can only hope that he survived to return safely to his bride.

We had come back almost ashamed, conscious of the enormous losses in equipment, lorries, guns and ammunition, all of which had been destroyed or rendered useless to the enemy. There were between two to three hundred of us off that craft, and we were all given a rapturous welcome as soon as we landed, indeed we were overwhelmed with offers of fruit, hot drinks, and sandwiches, as we were ushered onto waiting trains, which steamed off, one after another. We did not know to which destinations. Each station we stopped at, more and more refreshments were pushed through the open windows. Far, far more than we could cope with, and I regret to say the carriage floors were eventually ankle deep in offerings.

Such was the nation's relief and thankfulness that so many had already been snatched from the brink of utter disaster. Our destination turned out to be Matlock Hydro. The Padre, the Liaison Officer, La Batt, and I were treated as special guests. My first action was to dash to the telephone, and I rang up Rennie with the joyful news that, if she could manage to leave Clevedon, she could join me at the Hydro Hotel.

We had a wonderful week there, before leaving for home and the children at Clevedon. We had been feted and taken on drives around the Peak district. The Liaison Officer was surprised at the beautiful scenery. and remarked "Why do you English want to come to Switzerland, when you have similar lovely views in miniature here?" On the whole his outlook was depressing for he kept repeating, "If Germany had won the first war, then there would have been no second." His father was the Chief Commissioner of Police in Paris and with the Vichy Government now established, his view was extremely pessimistic, just when General De Gaulle was trying to rally all Frenchmen.

Our reunion as a family was far too short, as I was soon posted as Senior Medical Officer to a convoy for Abyssinia. There was so much that lad been left behind at Bexley, which was needed at

Clevedon, that I used the last twenty four hours of my leave to collect it. This meant driving from the West to Kent.

On arriving at Bexley, I fastened our trailer to the car and started to pack at once. Among other things were a gas refrigerator, super washing machine, various other household appliances and the children's toys etc. I started back at once and drove all night. What a mad thing to have done! It was early next morning when I reached Clevedon. Driving then, with dimmed headlights, was tiring, and I was exhausted when I reported for my medical before embarking with the convoy for Abyssinia. I was turned down on account of my cardiac condition. Exhaustion following first the Dunkirk episode, and then my mad rush to Bexley and back, had caused a temporary recurrence of my previous racing heartbeat. Stupidly the phrase "Dodging the column" kept repeating itself in my mind.

I soon recovered with rest, and we, as a family, all enjoyed the extra, so unexpected, respite. There was an excellent school at Clevedon, which Rennie arranged for our two girls, Elizabeth and Patricia, with their two cousins Bridget, and Janet, to attend, making a family foursome. The Headmistress was a remarkable and excellent teacher, and all four did well under her tutelage.

I was at last able to join in with a lot of their pony riding and walks with occasional trips to Weston-super-Mare. There soon followed a series of short postings to the Midlands. This was at the time, when those rescued from Dunkirk were sent to various centres, as the nuclei of new fighting units. The nation was spurred to tremendous toil in all vital sections of the war effort. All that was lost in France and Belgium had to be replaced, this meant not only fighting aircraft, but lorries, guns of all descriptions, ammunition and so forth. In addition, there was the replacement of losses at sea from the U-boats and sea raiders. These approached a catastrophic level in ships, seamen, and essential supplies of food and war materials.

This was the time of Dad's Army, and much as we enjoy today's amusing television episodes, let us not forget, that it was largely formed by veterans of the First World War, who knew personally from bitter experience, what war meant, yet who would have fought again, to the bitter end in support of their homeland.

My next posting was to Swindon, and I was billeted at the Bell Hotel. My duties were principally those attached to local M.I. rooms in the area. I was within easy distance of Clevedon, and so was able to spend more time with the family.

Opposite the Bell Hotel was a draper's shop. I was much taken with the appearance of a shantung silk outfit, which I thought would be ideal for Rennie. When I enquired about it, the Manageress showed great interest.

She wanted to know all sorts of what, to me, were technical details. Of course I was flummoxed.

Eager not to be wanting, the Manageress had all the assistants put on parade, in order for me to pick the one whose size and type of figure resembled Rennie's.

This 'identification parade' was great fun and provided an enjoyable interlude during this time of national anxiety. I feel sure the Manageress had seized this opportunity for a short relaxation of tension.

Amid the smiling participants, I had perforce to choose one. This, after some hesitation I did, and the chosen one was sent off by the Manageress to reappear in the two piece shantung suit to universal admiration, and to my pleasure when I thought of Rennie.

Rennie was delighted with the suit, the girls clapped their hands and the boys tried to be appreciative of the importance of this incident in a non-masculine world.

Meantime there was great activity as regarded training. Practice alarms of invasions by German paratroopers, were staged at strategic points, often in the early hours, kept us all on the 'qui vive'. Training went on day and night.

Units were suddenly ordered to other localities and my M.I. rooms were frequently changed. One day, I visited a wayside tavern which had housed the H.Q. of a company. In the courtyard I found two sacks. One was full of wheat flour, and the other of crushed oat flakes. It was beginning to rain, so I hurriedly asked the tavern keeper to take the two sacks under cover.

He refused saying that they were army property. I hastily covered the sacks with brown paper as a temporary protection. Then I tried other units, but all refused to take responsibility for the two sacks, as did the Police. I tried the local hospital without success. Everyone was afraid that they might he held culpable. This, when the country was so desperately short of food supplies.

Fortunately, the threatened downpour had not materialised, but the sky was dark and cloudy. I felt that I should have to get a move on to save the sacks from becoming soaked with rain. At the local ironmongers, I bought two galvanised iron bins. Returning to the tavern, just before the rain started in earnest, I got some help with lifting the sacks into the two bins, and placing them into my car. So far so good, and after more attempts to offload the many rations of flour and crushed oats, I decided to take them to Clevedon. One afternoon, as soon as it was possible, I set off. On the way down I began to have doubts as to whether I was acting in a questionable manner. As the miles passed, I began to feel ever more uneasy. What if I had an accident, how would the presence of army rations in my car look to an inquisitor?

It was nearly dark when I reached home. First I had a hurried consultation with Rennie about the bins. She said, "Bring them in," so I returned to the car and started to unload. Suddenly I was conscious of a large presence looming near. A policeman was standing beside me. All my recent misgivings rose accusingly to confront me.

****

"Can I help you with those heavy bins, Sir?" he asked. When I had recovered my equanimity, I gratefully accepted his offer. All went well and the two bins were safely carried into the kitchen. I heaved a sigh of relief. Rennie, who had prepared refreshments in time for my arrival, produced spanking hot cups of coffee. All three of us enjoyed this little respite. We thanked the constable for his timely assistance, and saw him on his way. After he left we embraced, with glee on Rennie's part, and relief and satisfaction on mine.

Rennie was able to save on her rations for many months, and as she had a large household to cater for, my dubious act of salvage proved its worth.

Back at Swindon, one morning there was an air raid alarm. As I entered one of the unit's parade ground to find a melee going on, a recruit was hysterical. He had been terrified as soon as the alarm sounded, and was being restrained physically by unsympathetic military police. My arrival on the scene was opportune, for with my earlier mental hospital experience, I realised that his condition needed investigation.

After careful assessment of his mental state, I referred him to the army psychiatric department. He was seen by a psychiatrist, who confirmed my opinion that he was definitely unfit for service and he was returned to civilian life. Nothing unusual about that apparently, but imagine my surprise when I received an invitation to dinner from one of the prominent tradesmen in Swindon. This was to express his gratitude and that of his daughter, who was engaged to the recruit, for my suggesting that he would be of more use as a civilian helping with the war effort, than in the army. I enjoyed that dinner!

It was now nearly mid summer and every day Hitler's invasion of the country was expected, but it was not until the tenth of July that the 'Battle of Britain' commenced, and the response of the R.A.F. was cautious. Radar stations were being constructed as fast as possible, and in secrecy. On the thirteenth of August Goering signalled 'Eagle

Day' and expected to achieve complete aerial supremacy in four days.

I had enough spare time to get back to Bexley, and do a little towards keeping the garden from going to ruin. It was at one of these times when I saw one of the huge air attacks on London. The sky seemed a mass of aircraft, and it was the distant drumming of numerous plane engines, increasing in volume, that made me look up. There seemed to be three tiers of aircraft, the lowest were probably bombers, above these were German fighters, as a protective shield, and higher still our own fighters.

This do or death aerial armada soon passed from my view. It was probably the first attack on London, and later I anxiously listened to the radio. In spite of the enormous damage inflicted on London and the docks, the losses of German aircraft far exceeded those of our own. Soon afterwards the so called 'Baedeker' raids took place. The tragic destruction of Coventry cathedral is well known.

Later Rennie and I had been on a shopping visit to Bristol. We were about to part, when, as I saw her on the bus for Clevedon the air raid sirens sounded. Almost the next minute the night sky seemed filled with German bombers. The noise was terrific. The screeching of dive-bombers and exploding bombs, pedestrians rushing to the air raid shelters formed only a background for the enormity of the anxiety both Rennie and I felt for each other as her bus and my car both left Bristol in opposite directions from the centre of the turmoil.

Rennie's bus travelled near the dock area. At times I could almost feel that the aircraft were so low, that they would scrape the car's roof. It was with relief that I at last realised, that the car was beyond the bombing area, and soon afterwards I heard the all-clear.

My anxiety for Rennie's safety was overwhelming, for she had been in the target area. Indeed the driver of the bus would not stop, though some of the passengers were troubled with travel sickness.

When at last I reached Swindon, I rushed to the telephone not expecting to get through. My relief was incredible, when Rennie herself answered. Our shared joy was one of profound thankfulness and humility.

Later we saw the now wrecked roads, along which we had so fortunately travelled safely.

It was only a few weeks later, that I received a 'permanent' posting to Carlisle. This was a blessing in one way but a disappointment in another. I had hoped for a specialist appointment, which had been promised. However a 'permanent' position, would enable Rennie to settle the question of the children's schooling. She arranged this and much else. Carlisle is a city of much appeal both for its history and its buildings. The park borders the river Aden, and we looked forward to a happy period there.

I suppose the lapse of time is responsible for my failing to recall the appearance of the building externally, that was to be my M.I. room. It was quite roomy and contained a ward and about a dozen beds. The floor had been recently concreted and the surface was powdery. The concrete had been made with very fine sea sand and a minimum of cement. Every time it was swept dust arose. I discussed how to deal with this problem with the N.C.O., a sergeant. He was at a loss what to do. I suggested an old remedy, which I had used elsewhere of old engine oil mixed with paraffin brushed over the whole floor, followed by polishing with a liberal amount of Mansion polish. He was horrified, and flatly refused to countenance such an idea without permission from 'Higher Authority'. I knew what that would mean, at least as regards wasted time.

I called at the local garage and asked for two gallons of old engine oil, two gallons of parrafin and a broad paint brush. I returned, but the staff refused to have anything to do with such a mad scheme.

"Very well," I said," I'll do the job myself."

I took off my tunic rolled up my sleeves and started to mix the ingredients. This was too much for my staff, who thought I was quite mad. However, they started to brush the oily mixture over the concrete. To their astonishment, it was at once absorbed, and the surface appeared a warm brown with very little smell, which disappeared within an hour.

Using Mansion polish on top, produced a result which they regarded with approval.

I now felt the loss of my specialist equipment, which had been abandoned at Dunkirk. On taking the matter up again, the response was, Could this not be a 'compendium'? For the loss of such an article, it was possible to claim up to £75. An old army regulation of the 18th century was unearthed on my behalf. I gladly received the compensation for the loss of my compendium. The start of the Michaelmas term was due in a few days, and our two daughters and elder son were, in their different ways, prepared to face this change in their lives, when I received notice that I had been posted to Colchester

Military Hospital, as Nose Ear and Throat specialist, with the rank of Major. So goodbye to my 'permanent' posting at Carlisle, and disruption of all the arrangements we had made. This was particularly upsetting for the children's schooling. Fresh plans had to be made as soon as possible. Fortunately, I had seven days leave, which was a great help. After explaining and apologising to the schools, and saying goodbye to the staff at the M.I. room, we left in our car for Bexley. Our caravan was waiting for us at St. Laurence, and towing the van, we sped on our way to Colchester. The weather remained fine, and on the whole the week's leave was a holiday, although rather an anxious time.

****

The Colchester appointment lasted for the best part of a year and from our family point of view, it was the best of the war years. Rennie returned to Clevedon, and the girls were able to resume their old school life. Waring, now aged six, started at a boys' school. This led to a rather amusing contretemps, when the girls' school had a holiday, but the boys' did not. This was beyond Waring's idea of what was right and proper. So he gave himself a holiday and stayed at home.

The headmaster enquired why Waring was not at school. He was quite shocked at the lad's behaviour, and took it upon himself to call round and sympathise with Rennie about the shocking conduct of her son. She, who had been quietly amused at Waring's reasoning, quickly responded by saying, "If you feel it was such a heinous offence, I will take him away at once." This totally unexpected reaction to the head's rather patronising approach, baffled him, and after a somewhat stuttered reply he left. No more was heard about Waring's truancy.

Having my own caravan home made a great difference. After my duties at the hospital, I was able to think what I could do for the family. I made a small workbench and spent evenings trying to make presents. Pencil boxes for the girls, a toy railway on a sheet of plywood 6ft x 4ft. for Morris, and a repeating machine-gun firing paper pellets for Waring. These efforts met with dubious success, but on the whole were a lot of fun. One day I was asked, as orderly officer, to check conditions at a large army cookhouse near Parsons Heath.

On the whole I was impressed by the care, general cleanliness and keenness of the staff. Two special points I always looked for - dishcloths - which tended to get tatty, and stationary objects - which were likely to become the home of insects and spiders. I had just finished the routine inspection when a large dish of beef dripping with brown gravy (of appetising appearance), was being carried out of the cookhouse.

"What do you do with that delicious looking dripping?" I inquired.

"It's to be burnt," came the reply.

I was shocked and asked "Why is it not eaten?"

The answer staggered me, "Nobody will use it." That turned out to be true. Neither the officers' mess, the sergeants', nor the troops, would consider bread and dripping as eatable.

My mind went back to the Dunkirk days when it would have been devoured with relish.

The idea of its destruction was so unacceptable to me that it followed the wheat flour and oats to Clevedon. It was certainly appreciated there. I tried to find ways of stopping such waste, but I had to give up.

At the hospital, one morning against the bright blue sky, I saw a German plane, apparently on reconnaissance. Then a Spitfire appeared out of the sun, and was apparently unnoticed by its quarry. We heard a distant crack of machine gun fire and the German plane crashed out of sight. The pilot managed to make a life saving landing, and he was admitted to Colchester Hospital severely wounded. He was the typical blond Nordic type.

He spoke English perfectly, having studied at Cambridge.

His first remark was "This is the nicest thing that could have happened to me." He was so different from the mental picture of what an enemy pilot should be in everyone's mind, that instead of treating him with cold, but faultless care, he was personally appreciated by members of the nursing staff. Quite a fuss was made of him, until he left for a prisoner of war camp. Was this a reaction from the heartrending anxieties of war?

I could not sympathise with this attitude, bearing in mind the memory of that youthful Spitfire pilot near Brussels. Once again I was able to help a local practitioner in the area, but petrol was severely rationed and I used my bicycle a lot. The R.E.M.E. had a repair depot nearby. One day I was asked to attend a casualty there. I had just about enough petrol to get there, and wondered how I should get back. After attending the casualty, I returned to the car and found to my astonishment that I had nearly a full tank of petrol.

The explanation was that when damaged vehicles were towed in for engine repairs. The petrol tanks had to be emptied on to waste ground. Another example of waste, but for me help. I was advised to leave my car there overnight anytime, when the 'fairies' would replenish my empty tank.

I was fast becoming a part-time disposer of waste!

Autumn soon came and went, and life in the caravan became austere. On frosty mornings during the winter I would wake to a sparkling frost on the inside of the roof. Fortunately I was connected to the main electricity supply.

My professional work at the hospital was very different from what I had been accustomed to at the children's hospital. Most patients were young and healthy. Emergencies were few and far between. Occasionally there would be cases of foreign bodies impacted in the gullet which had to be removed by oesophagoscpy. Examinations of hearing, tests of coordination, and non-emergency operations such as tonsillectomies.

During the spring and summer holidays, Rennie and the children were able to join me at Colchester. That meant finding extra accommodation. We had some enjoyable rambles and went bathing in the local river.

One day a circular from the war office arrived for all the M.Os., asking if they were willing to serve overseas, if required. This to me seemed unusual, to say the least. I filled up my form saying I was prepared to serve where I could be of most use. When I questioned my brother officers, they all replied that they would prefer to continue in their present jobs. The way of the authorities is peculiar to the war office. In a short time I was one of the very few M.Os, who had not been posted overseas! However, active preparations were in progress to prevent Germany using France's fleet, and overseas possessions against Britain. General de Gaulle was endeavouring to keep France in the war, by forming the Free French Army, which co-operated with the development of an underground resistance throughout the whole of occupied France. He hoped to carry on the war from North Africa and other French colonies.

Their humiliating defeat convinced many of the French that all was lost.

In contrast, in January, 1941, Britain started the New Year with her three fighting forces now refurbished, and determined to continue the fight against Germany to the end.

The Nation's self-respect was increased by the patriotic and enthusiastic speeches of Churchill, and by remarkable feats on the part of the Navy, the Army and the R.A.F. which led to victories by the Navy, the Army and the R.A.F.

The Navy established control of the Mediterranean, by destroying in action a large section of the Italian fleet.

The Army captured the Italian North African areas of Abyssinia Algeria, and Tripoli.

The R.A.F. destroyed the power of the Italian navy by the raid on Taranto, and secured air supremacy over North Africa. Meanwhile, steps had to be taken to prevent French overseas territories supporting the Vichy government, and permitting French warships being taken over by the Germans.

General de Gaulle did everything in his power, by means of personal visits, accompanied by representatives of the Royal Navy, to explain, that if the Free French and British Alliance was not allowed to add the French warships to the Allied side, action would be taken to render their use by Germany impossible, even if this meant bombardment by the Royal Navy. Loyalty to the Vichy government prevailed, and all French warships in overseas ports, which did not join the Allies, were destroyed, in spite of resistance by their crews.

Regrettably casualties were unavoidable.

The French colonies became anti-British. U-boats were sent to the Mediterranean, and to the West African coast.

British forces were widely deployed and needed reinforcement. Apart from the Middle East and North Africa, all areas on the West Coast of Africa under British protection were under threat from hostile Vichy French neighbouring colonies.

Convoys were sent to both areas. The U-boats were deadly, and British losses became heavy. One convoy with a hospital ship suffered severe casualties, including the hospital ship itself which carried personnel for the hospitals in the Gambia, the Gold Coast and Nigeria. The loss of life was catastrophic. The effect was felt in Colchester. I was suddenly posted overseas, but did not know my destination. There was a short period of leave to make arrangements, before I had to report to Leeds.

Rennie and the children were at Clevedon and I felt that the situation, as regarded them, was as satisfactory as was possible. I had to collect tropical kit, and turn up at the port of departure. Today I cannot recall which it was.

It was a large convoy, and we steamed due west out into the Atlantic. One wondered where we were going. It was amazing how this huge convoy was protected by the Navy and the R.A.F. We had been on this course several days, when the convoy split, our section turned south. The weather changed as we entered the trade wind area and we all enjoyed the warmth and sunshine. Our numbers included many medical and nursing personnel.

****

We all took advantage of the idyllic weather to sunbathe. One day a storm threatened, and as rain began to fall, the decks were soon deserted. I changed into bathing trunks, and had a wonderful time with the heavy tropical downpour cascading over me. After a short while others joined me, a little later the nursing staff appeared and there was much banter, laughter, and joking. I, who had been exposed much longer to the deluge, began to feel chilly, and withdrew.

As I left there was a sudden change, for with a clap like thunder, hailstones larger even than marbles crashed down. Safely below, I could hear screams and the rushing feet of the late arrivals scurrying for shelter. I was amused at the way some of the sufferers seemed to think I had planned it. Soon after that interlude, the convoy turned due east, and we were warned to be prepared to don life-jackets, as there was a possibility of U-boats being in the area.

The West African coast appeared, and at this point my memory fails me as to which port it was we called at first, although I know it was on the Gold Coast.

My first sight of Africa was a memorable one. The port had a long flight of very wide steps. These were crowded with Africans dressed in bright colours, descending and ascending, thus creating an ever varying tapestry of human figures.

Many small craft, including dugout canoes, were plying to and fro. We landed for a short time, and some personnel remained, having reached their destination.

We set out again, but were unable to proceed direct to our final ports, because the U-boat menace was now critical. We were diverted to Dakar, the port of French Senegal.

Surprisingly we were allowed ashore. There was a very different welcome from my previous experience of a French greeting. This was an atmosphere of cool correctness, evident in the way of the reaction to my purchase of a set of stamps at the post office. There was no hint of geniality. In fact I felt rebuffed. As I returned towards the quayside, I caught sight of a sailor spitting on the ground over which I had walked. Such behaviour was understandable, following the shelling and destruction of French warships which had not joined the Free French. However, no one cares to remain where he is obviously unwelcome, so I cut my visit short and returned to the ship. This was an example of the 'Perfidious Albion' opinion and will in due course be shown to change once more.

At last the U-boat menace was overcome and we sailed for our destination, which was The Gambia.

We landed by tender at Bathurst, and were taken by army vehicles to Fajara, the 55th. West African Hospital recently completed, and our future home in the West African Frontier Force for the duration of the posting.

It was the rainy season, and I never expect to experience another drive as depressing as that was for miles. The humidity was near 90°F. It was either pouring with rain, or misty, and perspiration streamed from every pore on the slightest exertion.

In the year 1588, England established a trading centre on a small island in the estuary of the Gambia river. This was the year of the Spanish Armada, when Queen Elizabeth, the first, was on the throne. The island was called St. Mary's and the capital was later named Bathurst, after one of the governors. The river Gambia was one of the main centres of the slave trade. In 1805 Britain abolished the slave trade.

It was due to the determination of Britain to end this loathsome traffic, that a British protectorate was established along the length of the river, with approximately 75 miles width of land on each bank. This was an international agreement between France and Britain. It paid no regard to the local African tribal areas. From the British viewpoint it was for trade, hence it was a protectorate, the tribes were at least nominally independent.

Eventually St. Mary's Island was connected to the mainland by Denton Bridge, on which were solitary railway lines for a railway to the interior, which was never built.

The 55th General Hospital had separate wards for African army troops and British. Both were treated equally.

I had been appointed as the Ear, Nose and Throat surgeon. I soon had other duties allotted to me. The first was Mess Officer, (I always seemed to land this job). Was it because I was a teetotaller? Another was O.C. gardens, which was a congenial one, but my knowledge of tropical agriculture was nil. Another job was 'Yaws' specialist, hence I was often dubbed 'Yours truly'. Finally a fourth one, inspector of the local gaol.

Having mentioned these extra duties, I will describe later details which arose connected with each of them.

These duties did not start at once, as there was a gradual take-over from the staff we were relieving.

As regards the officers' mess, the first thing I saw was cement dust. Here was the Carlisle problem once more!

The officers quarters, with the exception of the C.O's, who had a bungalow, were semi-detached bungalows. All were protected with anti-mosquito wire mesh netting.

We all had to be immunised against tropical diseases when in England, and in Africa we had to take anti-malaria tablets daily. These were yellow pills which gradually stained the skin. This process was so slow that we were unaware of its insidious development.

I was told that all the African 'boys' were thieves and that anything I valued, I should lock up. This seemed to me to be an intolerable nuisance. My batman really was a boy, about 16 years old, and I instinctively took to him. I told him, "If there is anything in my room you would like to have, please ask. If I can spare it, you shall have it, but never take anything without asking first."

One day he came to me in an agitated state, and said, "Please Psah, lock up sugar one time, or I chop him." This I did and I missed nothing all the time I was in the Gambia except for one incident.

Fruit was plentiful, oranges, bananas, pawpaws etc.

One Sunday I cycled to the Methodist Mission Church for evening service, and for a social get-together later. It was a very close and humid night.

I looked forward on my return to eating my last juicy orange. when I got back, dripping with perspiration, I found the orange missing. Next morning when my boy returned, I spun an exaggerated yarn of my journey back the night before tired out, parched with thirst, and with one possible hope of relief, the orange with which to ease my distress.

As I watched his face, he looked more and more conscience-stricken until tears rolled down his cheeks and he suddenly cried out: "I chop orange. Psah!"

"It is all right," I said, "That is 'forgot' now, Go for Baku, catch twelve orange, one time."

I gave him the money and off he went. He soon returned with twelve oranges, which he put on the table, with the money, and said "That is for dash," (Gift). He then produced another, saying "This be for orange, I chop." So harmony was more than restored!

I was puzzled by the use of the word 'Psah', when he talked to me. He explained the 'Psah' was because of my age, and was used instead of the customary 'Sah'. We live and learn.

****

The Africans appeared to me to exist in a world alive with evil spirits, 'debils', against which they tried to protect themselves with powerful 'jujus'. My boy said "If a man saw one special particular evil spirit, that man die, no one see him again." This unfortunate had to be alone when he saw the evil spirit. So I asked - "If the man was never seen again, how did anyone know he had seen the evil spirit?" This baffled him for a time, but then he replied "One man told just before he died." This blind belief in a world of debils, demons, and evil spirits was so ingrained in the mental make up of tribal beliefs, that even converts to Christianity were still tormented by these polytheistic phantoms.

The Church of England and the Methodists worked hard to allay these superstitious fears. In so many converts, the concept of a loving Jesus acted as a protective shield, covering, but not exorcising these hidden terrors. That is how the African mind seemed to me.

I was fond of cycling as far as the bush permitted and visited various villages. There was always a gracious greeting from the headman. On one occasion, I was asked if I would like to see the launching of a dugout canoe. I shall never forget this experience. The canoe was in a clearing, lying on its side. Facing the bottom of the dugout was a line of villagers with long canes. There was a sudden hush, then at a word of command all of them rushed to the canoe, and raising their canes they thrashed the dugout's side. Then in a trice the line of tribesmen hurried away as fast as they could into the bush. The headman explained to me that this was done to drive the evil spirits out of what was once the tree. The process had to be repeated again and again on both sides, before the actual launch, which unfortunately I had not enough time to witness.

Perhaps beating may have had some unknown practical benefit.

My bungalow sitting-dining-bedroom with the help of my 'boy' was at last fixed up to our joint satisfaction. He was very interested in the family photographs which I had arranged. He picked up Rennie's portrait and asked

"Dat be your wife, Psah?"

I replied "Yes."

"She be fine, Psah."

He paused to find an adequate adjective to add to his admiration. Then he said,

"She is past paraffin!" He then corrected himself and added "She be finer than that, Psah, She be past Denton Bridge!!"

One had to be careful what one did, or what one said, to the Africans. For should it be beyond their understanding, it would be attributed to 'magic'.

Before I grasped the danger of this, I was showing some minor conjuring tricks to one of the 'boys', who was a mess servant. I picked up a large citron. This fruit can be as big as a small melon, I covered it with a handkerchief, said "Acra-cadabra" and lo, when the handkerchief was removed, there was a lemon. I used the handkerchief again, and when I took it off, the lemon had vanished and only a pip was left. The boy yelled "Debel man!" Absolutely scared stiff, he would not listen to any explanation, and with shrieks of "Debel man," he jumped out of the mess window and fled.

About two weeks later, I was in a lorry on the way to Bathurst, when at a stop, he got in. As we gathered speed, he suddenly recognised me, and with a yell of "Debel-man," he leapt off the moving vehicle, fell, then gathered himself up and disappeared into the bush. I never saw him again, but I had learnt a lesson, and never again showed a trick to an African, without explaining how it was done first. I hoped to make amends by exposing magic. As O.C. gardens, I was fortunate to have an educated and astute Head Gardener. He was a tall African, always in a spotless white robe. Like all Africans he always hoped to say what would please his hearer, and never to let it be thought that a good idea was his own, but must be attributed to his audience.

Thus he would say, "Psah, You would like me to plant Pawpaw trees? It shall be done. You like plenty fine flowers to be in garden. That is good idea." So it would continue. I found myself credited with most exotic fruits that I had never heard of. Alas, my posting ended before these bushes and fruits brought forth their delectable produce.

So far, all these minor events took place during the early part of the tour, whilst the change of staff was in progress. Their final departure was heralded by a performance of "George and Margaret" in the hospital theatre. This was an excellent performance, and not only was it a triumphant end to their tour, but it was near Christmas, and so their farewell was full of hope for the future.

Among my brother officers were two who, because of our specialities, I naturally saw a lot of. One was the anaesthetist, and the other the surgical specialist. The surgical theatre was almost our domain. Other specialists such as the oculist, the pathologist, etc, made less use of the department. Operations except simple or local ones were avoided as far as possible. The humidity and tropical heat tended to aggravate the possibility of secondary infections. Nevertheless the theatre was in use nearly every day.

There was a rumour circulating about a recent secret leopard society sacrificial tribal murder. I never got to the bottom of this mystery, and enquiries I made among Gambians were quickly answered in such an evasive way, that I realised this was a forbidden area of tribal witchcraft and the underworld of hoodoo mysticism.

Some of our African personnel might be in some way implicated in this tribal religious cult. As the hospital's representative I was asked to inspect conditions within the prison, in case any of the hospital African personnel might be concerned.

It was to be a routine visit and no preparatory warning had been given.

Arriving at the prison, I rang the bell and the door was opened by the tallest African I had ever met. Like my gardener he wore a spotless white robe, this was crowned by a red Fez cap. I asked if I could see the Governor.

"He is out, Psah."

"May I see the Assistant Governor?"

"He is on leave, Psah."

I explained who I was and the purpose of my visit, and asked to see who was in charge. He drew himself up to his full height and replied,

"I am in charge, Psah. I am the Head Prisoner, Psah."

This amazing reply shook me. He invited me into the prison, and escorted me around the gaol. There were no army personnel there. After thanking him for his so meticulous assistance, I returned to the hospital somewhat bewildered.

I thought that it would be as well to ring the Governor's office and the situation was explained to me. This impressed me with the wisdom of British justice as applied in a protectorate.

The Governor had been faced with a difficult problem, for the area of the tribal territory in no way coincided with that of his jurisdiction. It would have been irresponsible to turn a blind eye to such a barbarous act as a ritual murder. Although they were not directly responsible, the Chief and some of his entourage were aware of what was taking place. Although against such ritual fetishism, they were powerless to interfere. From the British Governor's viewpoint, they were all guilty as accessories before and after the act. So that justice could be seen to be done, they were duly charged, convicted and sentenced to terms of imprisonment.

The Chief was made 'Head Prisoner' and he carried out his duties impeccably.

Gambians from the 'bush' looked upon a stay in prison rather as we do a holiday break. They had beds and excellent food and in no way felt aggrieved.

Nevertheless it was dinned into them that any further ritual murders would receive much severer sentences.

As far as I am aware, there were no further 'leopard' society murders within the Protectorate, at least not during my tour of duty.

It may be that I am biased, but what terrible disasters followed the withdrawal of British Colonial and Protectorate rule, within a few years of the end of the Second World War! Fortunately the Gambia has, so far, escaped the worst of these nightmares.

****

Now that the previous personnel had returned to the U.K., I felt free to attempt the treatment of the sandy concrete floors. It would obviously be sensible to start with my own quarters. I realised, if successful, there should be no obstacle to going ahead with the Mess and wards.

First, I visited the workshops, and was astonished at what I found being done. There was a saw-pit and men were cutting up huge trees into planks. Then old springs from motor vehicles were separated into their individual leaves. Each section was softened with heat, then divided into suitable lengths to make different tools. These were worked into blades for such articles as various wood planes, chisels, and other instruments. The cutting edges were case-hardened, and I saw large Jack planes, fitted with these cutting blades, at work. There was an unlimited supply of old engine oil, which was exceptionally darkened with burnt residue. This encouraged me to begin treatment of the soft sandy concreted floors. Paraffin was available in quantity.

My boy and I started on our bungalow floor, to the alarm of various semi-permanent residents, such as centipedes, spiders and small beetles. Other occupants, not unwelcome, were lizards, who inhabited the walls, and frogs which sat in the water of the tray of my keep-cool. This was formed out of a hollow building breeze-block, standing in the tray of water. So I could store cool drinks, and the frogs and lizards reduced the fly population.

It was a relief to be free of the dry sandy dust.

Before starting on the mess floors, I decided to pay a visit to the Mess kitchen, after all staff had left for the night. I was not surprised when I interrupted a congregation of cockroaches enjoying their midnight fun. So the kitchen became number one target. Just as I was about to begin, I was summoned by the C.O. I naturally thought this was to do with my contemplated onslaught on the mess floors.

He had sent for me however to discuss an urgent request from the French Governor in Dakau. Hereby is an astonishing story. Although the West African Frontier force had been organised in all British areas on the West African coast for purposes of defence, President Hoover must have arranged somehow for a small United States force to be sent to Dakau. Why? Was this to put a check on the influence of British colonialism? If so, it misfired in a curious way.

The American medical department had penicillin, but as supplies were limited, it was to be used only for U.S.A. personnel. The French Governor's young son developed an acute middle ear infection with early symptoms of meningitis. The French medical department urgently requested penicillin from the U.S.A. supply. This was refused, because of the ruling that it was for American personnel only.

In despair the frantic father rang the Governor in Bathurst. Could he help? He contacted the C.O. at Fajara, who called in the pathologist, and myself to discuss the situation.

Officially we had no penicillin. Unofficially the pathologist had managed to obtain a very small quantity, when in England.

He had kept it for an emergency. We discussed the chances of the boy recovering, if the penicillin could be flown to Dakau at once. The C.O. and Dr. Hemderson-Begg, the pathologist, flew to Dakau, and to our joy the small patient, after injection of the penicillin, made a complete recovery. As a result, there was a complete 'volte face' on the part of the French in Senegal. The British were no longer 'Perfidious Albion'. I wished I could have gone to Dakau to experience this change of heart.

Back to the Mess and the cockroach confrontation. When I explained what I wanted done, and this included the wrenching out of the cooking stove, I was told it was an impossible task, and the staff refused even to consider such a mad undertaking. As in Carlisle, I said, "Well if no one is going to help, I'll start on the job myself."

However, it was unreasonable to begin without making preparations for alternative cooking arrangements, for two or three days during the clearing, and then treatment of the dry absorbent sandy concrete floor. It turned out there was no lack of labour once the task was under way. The furniture had to be removed for a start, then came the effort of easing the cooking stove away from its permanent anchorage. At last it was freed and, as it was removed, there was exposed a huge medley of creepy-crawlies. They were promptly sprayed with D.D.T., swept up and destroyed.

The final rendering of the absorbent floor surface, with the mixture of old engine oil and paraffin plus D.D.T., was quickly completed, and the floor looked resplendent and without dust. The result exceeded all my hopes, as the Mess kitchen remained free from pests until the end of my tour.

The rest of the Officers' Mess was comparatively easy and the sandy dust no longer worried anyone.

My tour in the area was now nearing halfway, and I had some local leave to come.

A steamer trip up the river promised to be enjoyable. I decided to spend my leave exploring it. The Gambia river, at the mouth, is huge, and I watched the loading and embarking of a little crowd of Gambians with great interest. There were such a lot of chattering and excited children, with all their belongings piled high. As we cast off, a lengthy tirade was given by an important looking Gambian, who had risen from his seat amid a special group. This group was composed of the senior members of a tribe, together with their chief, and the orator was the Chancellor. His speech was an historical account of the tribe, and in addition he held forth about the personal prowess of the chief.

I could not understand a word of what was said, of course, but I could gather the gist of it. He repeated his speech at each river quay. These were made of wood, and appeared rickety to me, but they seemed efficient enough considering the numbers of folk, laden with goods, who frequented then. Our steamer heralded its coming with loud blasts on the horn, and from the ship's deck we could see the excited crowds running and scrambling, to greet the vessel.

Dugout canoes, which had flocked around the craft whilst at the quaysides, would paddle around us until the last moment. As we progressed up river we saw herds of hippopotami. They seemed quite graceful, as they swam quietly along. On the banks, crocodiles aroused themselves and went floundering into the water. I believe they are few in numbers today, and are almost an endangered species, so many having been killed for their hides. As we reached the higher parts of the river, we steamed between high banks which were terraced. This was most noticeable on the port side. This area was called the monkeys' parliament, and I was told, that at a certain time of the year, monkeys gathered on these terraces and a huge 'palaver' took place.

Unfortunately, my memory fails me when I try to recall all I saw on this memorable up-river trip, the notes I made at the time have not survived.

Summer, 1944, and all in the Gambia were awaiting 'D' day, with a mixture of enthusiastic optimism and anxiety. When would the long awaited invasion of Nazi occupied France take place? Memories of the Dieppe raid with its heavy casualties still lingered in our minds.

Uncertainty of time and place persisted, and everyone was in a state of expectancy. Eventually, it was decided to hold a sweepstake as to when the attack would take place. Each member of the Mess was to write his guess of the date and enclose it in a sealed envelope, to be opened as soon as news of the landing was heard. Everything was so hush-hush that we could only guess.

I had made friends with a French merchant, who was an ardent supporter of De Gaulle, and I mentioned the sweepstake to him. He laughed and said "I can tell you the exact date it will take place. Officially it will be on the 5th of June, but actually not until the 6th." I laughed, and asked "How on earth, could you know and be so definite?" His reply staggered me. "I can tell you in confidence that I am a member of the 'Resistance', he said. "In fact I am their representative in the Gambia. The date of the invasion is definite."

"That is hard to believe" I demurred, "for hopes of success rely mainly on the element of surprise." He smiled and responded:

"The Germans have been told so many certain dates, one more could not alter the situation." I wondered, should I believe him? At any rate I wrote the 6th of June on my piece of paper, put it in an envelope, sealed it, inscribed my name on the outside and handed it in. I then began to have doubts, if my French friend was correct, then it would be unfair to compete. I solved this dilemma by saying I had learnt the actual date, and therefore withdrew from the draw, but there was my forecast for confirmation later. It proved to be correct, in spite of the official claim that it should have been the 5th of June.

Some time before 'D' day our C.O. was invalided home, and, as the next senior, I took over the command. If I had continued as C.O. for three full months, I would automatically have been promoted to Lt. Col. and have continued as O.C. The last day dawned, and almost at the eleventh hour a replacement C.O. arrived, just in the nick of time for the establishment.

****

In a way I felt disappointed, but on the other hand, my knowledge as regards infantry training was that of the 1914 era, I would have been at a complete loss as to how to form 'Threes'; and to order 'Form fours' would have created chaos!

Still, I would have appreciated the rise in pay.

However, in spite of my fear of creating havoc as O.C. on official parade, that very thing happened when the A.D.M.S. for the W.A.F.F. decided to inspect the 55th hospital, and to my alarm it fell to my lot to organise the parade. I did not mention my misgivings to the new C.O., but appealed to our company officer, who was not a medico, for help. He was amused, and perhaps hoped for some entertainment on the great day. For he took the attitude 'It will be all right on the day!'

So it turned out. Fortunately the three companies formed threes automatically, and I was able to lead my gallant troops past the saluting dais, on which the A.D.M.S. and our C.O. were ensconced (I think the company officer had been more helpful than he had led me to believe).

Soon after this episode, I was asked to be a member of a Court Martial, which was convened to try one of our African troops, who was charged with the attempted shooting of his officer. The bullet had pierced the officer's hat, but fortunately he was unharmed. The accused was a man of the highest repute, but there seemed no other possible decision but guilty. The defendant's plea that he was aiming at a bird, and had no intention of harming the officer, seemed unbelievable.

The Padre spoke up, however, to the relief of every member present.

He explained how the incident had occurred. The accused had no knowledge of ballistics. To him, the rifle was a magical weapon which killed what it was aimed at, and if it missed, the bullet would travel no further and drop to the ground.

The bird had flown on a collision course towards the officer, and he had shot in order to protect him.

Other African troops were questioned, and ignorance of ballistics where firearms were concerned was found to be widespread.

The defendant was found to be innocent, thanks to the Padre's timely and brilliant interpretation of the African mind.

The surgical specialist generally called at my bungalow for a cup of tea in the afternoon. This was possible, because Rennie had sent me a small electric stove, which was a marvel. A simple contraption, it would boil a kettle, toast, bake or roast. One afternoon he called in great distress as his cycle free-wheel no longer ceased free-wheeling. What to do about it, we discussed over our tea. Then we set about the bicycle. After removing the rear wheel, I dismembered the free-wheel, and found that the cams were shaped like a half moon. One end of each cam was worn, but the other not. Reversing the cams solved the problem, and the cycle once more was its old self. Often, we would go down to the beach at Fajara for a swim. We were fortunate at the Gambia, as there was a reef along the shore which was impassable for sharks, and we could swim in safety.

One afternoon, I was swimming parallel with the shore when Dick, the surgical specialist, suddenly saw not one 'Robo' swimming, but three! He rubbed his eyes and there were still three.

Meanwhile I was using the overarm side stroke when to my alarm, I saw a dorsal fin close to me. My first thought, a shark had managed to get within the reef, just as I was feeling terrorised, I saw a brown eye regarding me, and as I was in comparatively shallow water I stood up. To my surprise, there was another brown eye watching me on the other side. Then as it appeared to me, the pair of dolphins flourished their tails as though saying "So you are all right", and away they swept so gaily through and over the waves. Although snorkels were not yet available, I liked to swim under water and open my eyes to see as much as I could. There were always currents of some sort, and semi-submerged objects often appeared. Another moment of alarm happened one day, when I negotiated my way round a rock, and suddenly rushing towards me was a huge apparition with numerous waving arms or tentacles. It looked enormous, and as it crashed into me, I realised it was the bole of a palm tree, and the tentacles were decaying fronds.

What I found to be in truth the most unpleasant part of bathing in the tropics, was when the tide had receded, and I had to run over the hot sand to reach my clothes.

One evening on the way to the mess for dinner, a small white and black kitten accosted me with a "Meow."

"Meow to you," I replied, and thought no more of the matter. This happened again the next day, and on the third occasion, the kitten suddenly jumped from a small tree on to my neck and uttered yet another "Meow." It had adopted me, and became another resident of my bungalow. Amazingly it did not object to the other tenants. Certainly the kitten knew its own mind for each morning it would accompany me to the Mess. As I reached the door it would climb into the small tree, and when I left it would jump again onto my shoulder. True I was not carrying a pack on the end of a staff, otherwise I would have expected to hear the bells of Bow, a tropical version of Dick Whittington.

It was now approaching the last quarter of the year and as the floor of the Mess sitting room was now smooth and attractive, the Mess decided to have a dance. The nursing staff and some of the mission staff and British residents from Bathurst were invited. I felt sorry for our nurses, for by regulations, in order to avoid being bitten by mosquitoes, they had to wear long white boots which laced up well above the knees, not the most appropriate footwear for dancing. It was an enjoyable evening, especially as the R.A.F. dance band gave of their best. All went well, supper was a success, and so would the finale have been, but when supplies of the available alcoholic drinks were nearly exhausted, some of the younger enthusiasts raided the pathological laboratory for absolute alcohol to add to the loving cup. Unfortunately, this beverage had already been augmented by a quantity of native palm wine of unknown potency. The effect of this concoction was almost indescribable.

Fortunately the nurses would have none of it. Those officers who did, were soon seized with projectile vomiting, and became almost unconscious. Fortunately, there were no fatalities. Several pairs of dentures had been ejected with the vomiting. Next morning, their owners, when they had recovered sufficiently to see straight, had the task of sorting them out. The Mess floor, I am glad to say, stood up well to these ravages, and I had no complaints from the owners of the dentures about unsavoury flavour from the paraffin or old engine oil! Soon there was the advent of Christmas to prepare for, and as O.C. Mess, I had to do what I could as regarded decorations. The long tables with seats each side were a problem. There were plenty of flowers for festive effect, but no containers. I was undoing a roll of cotton wool, when I realised the wrapping paper was a perfect shade of Wedgewood blue. I got the idea of covering empty milk tins with this paper, and then making cut-outs from white paper of Greek figures. These were easy to mass produce, and when stuck on the paper covered tins, formed imitation Wedgewood vases. The effect, when they were filled with flowers added a touch of floral gaiety to the tables. The Mess cooks excelled themselves by conjuring up delicacies to whet everyone's appetite.

Our Christmas dinner, with all the nursing staff present, was a memorable and happy one, as we included toasts to all our relations and friends at home, and elsewhere in the forces. It fell to my lot to produce the next show, and I decided that instead of a straight play, a variety performance would be easier to stage, offering more opportunities for staff to display their talents.

The N.A.A.F.I. came to the rescue in an unexpected way. The stock of boiled sweets had suffered from the humidity and tropical heat. They had become candified. I wondered if they could be coated with tropical chocolate, and so make attractive chocolates. This is where Rennie's stove came in. I melted the tropical chocolate and dipped the candified sweets, separately into the hot mixture, then set them out in rows on paper. The result, while not up to the most exacting standards of confectionery, were certainly edible, and would be a surprise. The sergeants and some of the nurses gave a charming dancing display with vocal embellishments. One rapturously received and which still lingers in my memory was "After the ball was over." After a lapse of nearly fifty years, it is not easy to recall the wide variety of talent which came to light.

My turn consisted of a conjuring trick. I visited the workshop once more and made a box large enough to accommodate a person. It was similar to the Princess Lotis's treasure chest of "The Egyptian Dream." Two members of the audience were asked to come on stage. I got into the box, they replaced the lid and secured it with ropes round front and back, also on both sides. As they returned to their seats, I appeared at the back of the hall, reached the stage, freed the ropes, raised the lid. When lo and behold! ...the recent performers, one by one, appeared out of the box, bearing a tray of chocolates for distribution among the audience.

****

Although the Gambia is mainly low lying country bordering the Gambia river, there are some hardwood trees. These consist of quite valuable timber for veneers. One specimen is locally called 'Iron wood', it so hard. I had three or four specimens of it about 5 x 4 x 2 inches. They were given to me by a Gambian who called at the hospital, hoping to sell locally made bags, wallets, and carvings. Some of these carvings were remarkable. The local craftsmen would sit on their haunches, whilst they gripped the piece of wood they were carving between their feet, using their toes almost as accessory fingers.

The first Christmas I was at the hospital, there was a demand at the hospital for Christmas cards, but none were available. It suddenly occurred to me, why not try to make a woodblock engraving from one of these pieces of 'iron' wood?

The result was no work of art, but it did supply a want and several hundred were roughly printed, one by one, by hand. One or two pieces of the hard wood were spoilt in trials, one piece looked as though some fierce beast had bitten off a chunk. When the 'bagman' called again, I showed him that piece first, with the words, "It be fine, fine, chop. Watch me while I pretend to chop him one time." I palmed it, then took up another piece, exchanging it for the palmed specimen and pretended to take a bite out of it.

When he saw that I had apparently bitten off a piece of 'iron' wood, his look of fearful amazement caused me hurriedly to repeat the performance, this time so that he could see how it was done. He then spent some time trying to do the trick himself.

I was relieved that no hint of magic was present. I hoped he might know the lad I had scared previously with a similar trick, and explain the so-called 'magic'.

A private sawmill had been started before the war, to supply this hard timber. The manager had attracted an efficient work force by giving the workers a super lunch of tinned salmon. The supply of salmon ran out and with the U-boat blockade, it was impossible to get further supplies. Fortunately, the manager was able to procure a quantity of corned beef, which came from one of the South American states.

Soon after his workforce diminished, and he was at his wits end. He asked the Chief to see him, to enquire why the workers were boycotting his mill!

The Chief replied that when the men had fish for lunch and the cans all had the picture of a salmon on the outside, "That be fine," but, when the cans of meat arrived with a picture of a Negro herdsman on the outside, the chief said "My men no agree for dat."

It took a lot of persuasion to convince the workers that there was no fear of them being 'canned'.

There were regular entertainments. Cinema shows in the open air were favourites not only with the units from the neighbourhood, but for the Gambians, including many from the bush. Cars could drive up and their occupants had no need to dismount. The screen was large and could be viewed from both front and back. From the back the pictures were like mirror reflections. Curiously enough, the Africans, even those from the bush, seemed to accept this as just another 'White Man's 'know-how', and did not attribute these moving pictures with voices to 'Debels' or evil spirits.

They were not without other effects however, for when I attended the Mission one afternoon, a number of the senior girl pupils were having a natter outside the school. Listening and keeping my ears alert, I heard them addressing each other by the Christian names of popular film stars.

One especially amusing remark which I overheard was, "No Marlene, dear, you cannot possibly wear that"

"Why not Gloria?"

"Because you are a blonde, Marlene."

I could see a slight lightening of Marlene's youthful smooth coffee hue, but I think they were playing me up! Peals of laughter and giggles followed this conversation. What was true was that they had all been christened after film stars. One of the teachers from the mission appeared, the giggling ceased, and the chastened group then meekly dispersed. As well as cinema, there were horse races, and among other sports, hockey was a favourite game. I was selected to play for the Cape Casuals at outside left.

There was a competition, and I recall that the final was between the Cape Casuals and the R.A.F. The two finalists were neck and neck, when suddenly the ball was passed to me, I feinted, then centred, and our centre forward scored the winning goal. Our nurses were there in strength, and in a mood of exuberant puffed-up pride, I glanced in their direction expecting to be admired.

What I saw was intense disappointment, for they all wanted, and expected, their darling lads of the R.A.F. to win.

It was about this time that my neighbour, in his semi-detached bungalow, was posted elsewhere. Naturally I was anxious to learn who would be taking it. No one seemed to have any idea. So I dropped a hint in the Mess, to the effect that I was thinking of taking a correspondence course on the trombone. A day or two later the Pathologist asked me, "Robinson, is it true you are learning to play the trombone by correspondence?" Relieved to discover the truth, I replied "Are you to be my next door neighbour? If so you need have no worry on that score."

Apparently there had been some difficulty about his vacating his present room, and he had been keeping mum. I was glad to welcome him as a future neighbour, and assured him that he need have no fears of being disturbed by the raucous screech of a trombone in the early hours.

Soon afterwards there was an outbreak of sleeping sickness among the animals in the Gambia. An order for the immediate slaughter of all pets in the hospital was issued.

I had become very attached to my kitten, and could not bear the idea of the destruction of such a trusting and affectionate animal. It was not as if I had adopted it, it had adopted me. I discussed with my new neighbour the possibility of taking the kitten to a place miles away and leaving it there. The pathologist thought that might be tragic for the animal. Two days later, I found the kitten dead, apparently having died during the night.

Nothing more was said but I think the pathologist had solved the dilemma for me.

So far it must appear that I did very little actual medicine. Certainly there was very little to do as regards my speciality was concerned.

However, although my knowledge of tropical diseases might been nil when I arrived, it rapidly increased, because the hospital out-patient department was available for the civilian Gambian population. There were numerous cases of Yaws, Leprosy, and parasitic diseases to treat.

Yaws is an ailment caused by a spirochete, similar to syphilis, but is spread through walking barefooted, when the spirochete invades the sole, and eventually spreads. Treatment is similar to syphilis and requires regular intravenous injections. Sometimes, there would be thirty or more patients awaiting injections. In obese subjects, the veins are often difficult to locate with dark African skins.

Intravenous needles were sterilised in boiling oil, as many as fifty at a time in rows, then used again in sequence.

Sterilisation was absolute. Nowadays, it is 'the throw away age' and a needle is only used once.

It was about this time, when my tour had already exceeded the usual eighteen months, that I became anxious about the health of the C.O. He showed a tendency to become introverted, and sat at night in the Mess alone. He sought relief in my opinion by consuming alcohol but never appeared other than sober.

Nevertheless, I am sure that his moroseness affected his judgement, for late at night, he would suddenly call an emergency parade of all hospital staff. This would be reasonable occasionally, but it became a more and more frequent happening. Many of the African staff on day duty would return to their homes to sleep. Africans appear to be heavy sleepers. Many would miss these night calls.

They naturally felt personally aggrieved when charged with being 'Absent from parade'. They were furious when penalised. I heard definite threats of an assassination plan.

My information was such that I felt action must be taken to prevent matters getting worse. The C.O. dismissed the threat as nonsense. The other officers agreed with me about the seriousness of the situation, but were unwilling to take any active part officially.

I rang the A.D.M.S. in Nigeria and asked for advice. I was told this was a delicate situation, but that it would be dealt with in due course. It certainly was. First it was pointed out that I had been nearly two years on tour, and that I was overdue for return to the U.K., and secondly, action was to be taken with regard to my report.

I sometimes wonder how long I would have remained in the Gambia, but for this difficult predicament.

I was seen off by the C.O., who was most cordial and full of good wishes. I learned later that he soon followed me. All of the officers of my tour had already left some time before, and it was with delight that I welcomed the prospect of my own return.

I flew from Yum Dum airport to the Gold Coast. This flight was very bumpy, as there were heavy turbulent cloud formations. For some time the pilot when near our destination circled and circled the area. Suddenly he spotted a small gap in the clouds with a clear view of the ground below, then he dived down and we could see the airport.

The touchdown was perfect, and we disembarked full of admiration for our pilot and his aircraft, a Dakota.

****

There was no urgency for the moment, after arriving at the airport, I had time to check on my baggage Two cases had been sent on by sea, yet only one had arrived.

The recent happenings at the hospital had had the effect of taking my mind off minor personal affairs. Now that I had time to consider my future position, I was wondering what was awaiting me in England. To my surprise my financial state was better than I expected. This was due to the overseas allowance which had accumulated.

Most of my colleagues had found the allowance insufficient. There was one explanation and that was the cost of alcoholic drinks.

My French friend in Bathurst had helped me to select various presents to take home. These included dress lengths and other things only obtainable at home with clothing coupons. I was assured that the missing case would be sent on in time. Then I went aboard my transport for home.

Farewell West Africa!

The U-boat menace was still much in evidence. The threat was such that the ship had to wait in the outer basin of Gibraltar. My friend, Gerald Rudolf, was stationed there and apart from the chance of seeing him, the fortress was of interest to me, as my great-grandfather was buried there. He was barrack-master general and died in 1816. Unfortunately no shore leave was allowed, as we were due to leave at any time.

I was disappointed not to be allowed ashore, but on the other hand, I was fortunate to see this outpost of the Empire when I did.

My first sight of Gibraltar was a dazzling wonder. The rock was sparkling with ice and frost, it shone like a gigantic jewel scintillating in the rosy rays of dawn. A barely perceptible corona of morning mist covered the harbour in which ships of war and supply waited expectantly.

We left within twenty four hours, and were warned to carry our life-jackets with us. Some officers would not sleep in their bunks but kept awake or dozed during the night. I chose my bunk, having practised finding my boat station with my eyes closed. Apart from that I have very little recollection of the journey from Gibraltar to our home port. In fact I cannot now recall which one it was. Every detail of the journey by rail to Kendal is lost in the joy of once more being united with Rennie and our family.

Rennie's uncle, Finn Payne, and his wife, Francis, had opened their home to Rennie and the children, when St. Laurence was damaged by the flying bomb. They had been so kind and welcoming to my family, and now extended their warm and affectionate hospitality to me. We shall never forget their generosity and kindness.

Aunt Francis had a wealth of North Country sayings. One which she would often use, rousing herself was "This and worse will never do, this and better may do!"

During this period of the war, forests of conifers were being planted among the hills of the Lake District. This distressed Uncle Finn, who pointed out how many of the loveliest views were being lost.

My leave seemed so short, and soon I received a new posting to Shaftesbury, as the Ear, Nose and Throat specialist there had been posted overseas. However, he made a point of calling on me to ask if I would object to having an alternative post, as he was in a critical phase of some research, which he hoped to complete. I was quite willing to move, but on condition that it was not overseas.

My new appointment was attractive, and I very much doubted whether my predecessor would succeed in his hope of returning. Whilst awaiting the result of his application, I agreed in the event of his appeal being granted, to act as his locum tenens. All went well for a few days, then one morning, I had a call from the operating theatre. This was an urgent petition from the anaesthetist, to the effect that he found it impossible to intubate a patient's larynx, therefore he entreated the E.N.T. surgeon to try, as the operation had to be done at once. I was flabbergasted, and. quite apprehensive, for the simple reason that anaesthetists must pass laryngeal tubes far more frequently than an E.N.T. surgeon. I set off for the theatre, when I entered, I felt that the tension and anxiety of the 'new boy' must be obvious. The theatre staff were looking exhausted, and on the floor were scattered laryngeal tubes of different sizes. Everyone, except the patient, who was snoring on the operating table, looked at me.

There was a hurried explanation of the patient's sensitivity, which resulted in violent rejection of all efforts to intubate his larynx.

At that moment, I seemed to hear the gypsy's voice of years ago, saying "You see with your fingers." Having 'scrubbed up', I took the laryngeal gag, with its tongue depressor, out of the patient's mouth, replacing it with a simple 'Doyen's'. Then I selected a laryngeal tube of suitable size, lubricated it, and passed it into the patient's mouth, at the same time visualising, with my fingers, the contours and shape of the oral cavity and pharynx. I sensed the epiglottis and detected the vocal cords. Pausing until the cords opened as he took a breath, I slipped the tube between them into the larynx. The patient gagged a little, but he breathed through the tube. I assured the anaesthetist and surgeon all was now well, and left them to it.

I had been in the theatre for five minutes at the most. When I got back to my own department, there to my surprise was the specialist, whose job I had taken over.

His application had been successful, and I had been appointed to the hospital at Moretonhampstead, Devonshire.

My stay at Shaftesbury had lasted only a fortnight, and certainly of the two, Devonshire, with Spring now so near, had great appeal.

I telephoned the hospital at Moretonhampstead, and left next day. I had no idea, at the time, I was on my way to my last posting in the army.

The hospital was a wartime conversion of a first class hotel. It had been built by W.H. Smith, originally as a private residence.

The site, on the edge of Dartmoor, was one offering boundless opportunities for exploring Devonshire.

Before the war, the German ambassador, Count Von Ribbentrop, had been a guest at the house. He was reported as saying that he would make it his private residence when Germany had won! It was now March, 1945, and Germany was reeling from attacks by the Allies on all fronts.

Fortune favoured me, for I was offered the lease of a large cottage, beautifully furnished. This was too good a chance to miss, so I rang up Rennie and we decided to accept the offer. Soon we were all enjoying, not only the comforts of such a super cottage, but had the opportunity of exploring the moor in spring. On one occasion, we came on a breathless vista of sparse woodland carpeted with bluebells. As we emerged from the trees, before us was a meadow, sloping luxuriantly down to a murmuring stream, which was spanned by an old packhorse bridge. The profusion of bluebells, augmented by the rich fertility of the soil, was such a wondrous sight that we were overcome by nature's lavish beauty.

Work at the hospital was largely routine, with regular operations sessions and few out-patients.

On May 5th, 1945, V.E. Day, Germany surrendered, and the war in Europe was over.

The Nation's rejoicing at the prospect of reunion with loved ones and of better times to come, after years of anxiety, hardship, and the terrible casualty lists, which those who have not lived through that period one can only imagine.

At Mortenhampstead, everyone at the hospital joined in the national exultation.

Later on that V.E. night, when alcohol was flowing, the sight of normally staid staff hilariously playing bowls in the lovely oak panelled hall, to the detriment of the woodwork, was distressing to me. I could not bear to watch this senseless vandalism and retired to our temporary home.

At this time I had quite a list of personnel awaiting operations. True they none of them were of immediate urgency, but I had expected to deal with those cases already arranged fairly promptly. That is however not the service custom, dates are all important. Today one is in the army, tomorrow one is once more a civilian.

As a family we were delighted at the prospect of returning to Bexley, and resuming our lives from where we had left off, though not without some regret at leaving Devon. We determined to have future holidays in the area, and especially to see again that bluebell fairyland.

That is 48 years ago, and now I cannot fully recollect how we managed at first. St. Laurence was not fit to occupy and was in a dangerous condition. All contents had been removed, and were in store at Long Reach miles away.

Dr. Stewart, who had kindly looked after the practice during the war, offered me the use of his surgery, as a temporary measure.

One of my first visits was to the Children's hospital at Sydenham. The welcome I received was enthusiastic, and I was told that I could resume my pre-war duties as E.N.T. specialist.

Imagine my chagrin, when I learnt that my pre-war appointment was now filled by two surgeons, wartime emergency appointees at a salary of £800.00 p.a. each. I could resume my voluntary appointment, but it could not be classed under the heading of 'Emergency', as the war was over, and would remain 'voluntary'. My position was difficult, as if I resumed my full pre-war activities, it would leave the other two surgeons to do little or no work. On the other hand, the prestige of Honorary Surgeon in a Voluntary Hospital was such, that I had to pause for thought before deciding what to do.

Among other problems, there was still the remainder of the mortgage on St. Laurence to be paid. The Building Society agreed to wait until the war damage to the house had been assessed and paid by the Government.

My pre-war car, the Humber-Snipe, was still retained by the garage in lieu of payment.

First things first; a careful valuation of the bomb damage to the house was made and duly presented. It was cut by half, with the unofficial explanation that all claims for bomb damage were over estimated. However, it paid off the outstanding mortgage. From the security of army service, I was now floundering in a sea of confused civilian chaotic uncertainty.

****

Rennie and I considered the position; first, as regarding the practice. The changes in population, due to the war, had at the very least reduced my number of patients to less than half. Many of the others had been treated by brother practitioners for four years and any young children were, understandably, averse to a doctor new to them. There were the two branch practice houses, occupied by caretakers on a permanent basis. One of Hitler's refugee doctors had started in practice close to one of them.

Our children's education was another problem.

Fortunately Elizabeth had matriculated, and applied to the University of London to start training for medicine. Her application was rejected, as there were so many former medical students returning from war service, and they had priority. She was advised to apply again in two or three years. She was very disappointed but decided to take up radiography, and started her training.

Paddy was still at school, as were the two boys, Waring and Morris.

Our caravan, which had remained in the front garden of St. Laurence, appeared almost unaffected by the blast from the flying bomb. On closer inspection, however, the body had burst outwards, and then settled back in position. It was a write-off. It fetched £30.00 as the chassis was undamaged.

A few weeks after my return to Bexley, I had an urgent call from an old patient of mine, she lived near one of the branch surgeries. Would I call urgently to see her child?

As soon as I saw the little girl, I was horrified to see what I had never seen before, the dreadful 'Risus Sardonicus' of lockjaw. Such an advanced case of tetanus was probably hopeless. However, I gave her anti-tetanic injection of serum, and rang the hospital at Sydenham.

There was a private bed available, and I took her there in my car to save time. On arrival, I was told that the emergency surgeon was already operating elsewhere, and would I act on his behalf?

The history of the case was: some days previously the child had been playing near the railway, when she fell, and drove a piece of iron deep into her calf muscles.

Her parents took her to the refugee doctor, who stitched up the wound, bandaged it, and sent her home.

Then followed a struggle to save the child. This meant, first, a general anaesthetic, then, opening up the wound, flushing it with peroxide, and cutting out all damaged tissue, eventually leaving the wound open.

For two days and nights the convulsions were appalling. It was necessary to keep her under sedation and re-anaesthetising her during the worst spasms.

Finally on the third day she improved and slowly recovered. Her parents paid for the private room at the hospital. They took legal advice and decided to sue the doctor.

He rang me up to ask for my advice. He said "I did not recognise the tetanus when I saw it. I thought that the child would not open her mouth. I damaged some of her teeth when I looked at her throat. What do I do now?"

He was a member of the same defence body as I was, The Medical Defence Union, so I told him to seek their advice.

I sent a bill to the parents, I forget the amount but it was under £40. To my amazement, I later received a letter from the Union, suggesting that I waive my fee, as the other doctor was a brother practitioner! This struck me as intolerable, and I replied that I had probably saved the doctor from a charge of malpractice, which, but for my action, would have led to much more serious charges. I expected to be paid for my work, especially as the child had been admitted as a private patient. The union duly paid my fees.

Meanwhile, the parents decided to sue the doctor for damages. They had a clear case, but on consulting a solicitor, they were informed that any damages would naturally be placed in trust for their daughter. When they found that they could not use the money, they dropped the case. They were Italians, which may have influenced them in some way.

To my indignation, the doctor concerned telephoned me a week or two later, and said that he understood I might have to sell my practice. If so, he would be prepared to make an offer. My refusal to consider such a suggestion was appropriately abrupt.

I forget the amount of leave on full pay the army gave me, but it was for a period of some months. This had sufficed to enable me to carry on for some time, in spite of the reduced earnings from the practice.

Also there was the prospect of the National Health Service being introduced in the near future.

One day, I returned home to discover that Rennie had had a dreadful experience. I have mentioned that the council had temporarily provided a not completely finished house for us. There was a large manhole, with a cover, in the centre of the way into the front garden. Rennie had stepped on it, and it had collapsed. She fell through, but fortunately spread her arms out in time, and came to a stop, her feet still not touching bottom. Most fortunately a passer-by saw her dangerous predicament and managed to extricate her.

She was in bed when I got home, badly bruised and suffering from shock. I at once reported the matter to the council, and that death trap was put right. I say death-trap because a similar accident happened to a man in the area, and he was swept away into the main sewer and drowned.

I was advised to sue the council, which put me in a quandary.

We had been grateful for the temporary shelter, and I doubted the wisdom of taking legal action.

About this time I saw an advertisement in the The British Medical Journal for an Oto-rhino-laryngologist in Leicester.

On enquiry, I found the duties were mainly in the County at Markfield, Hinckley, plus sessions at the Royal Infirmary, Leicester.

Salary would be on a sessional basis, and largely increased in comparison with my meagre income at Bexley.

I applied for the post, and at the same time obtained the counsel and help of the B.M.A. with regard to selling my practice.

I attended for interview and was appointed. The B.M.A. found a purchaser for the practice. He came to Bexley for a period of introduction to the patients.

All went well, and I was able to replace the caravan, and have the new engine fitted to my Humber Snipe.

On my retirement from the Children's Hospital, Sydenham, I was appointed : Hon. Consulting Oto-rhino-laryngologist.

My new appointment started late in the year. Accommodation was impossible to find at first. As a temporary measure I sought out a farmer at Thurlaston, who willingly allowed me to put the caravan on his land. As the caravan had six berths, it could at a pinch accommodate the whole family, until a suitable house became available in Leicester.

Both our daughters were away. Elizabeth was training as a radiographer, and Patricia vas training in nursing at Great Ormond Street Children's Hospital.

Little did we dream that the winter of 1946 would be the severest for years. However we were snug and comfy. At first I had no trouble travelling to and from Leicester and the other hospitals. Later we were cut off by drifts of snow. The main roads were kept open, but the minor road to Thurlaston was impassable for weeks.

Prior to the final blizzard, which cut off our village and farm.

Paddy had a period of leave due, and I drove to London to fetch her. It had started to snow and I found myself driving through one of the worst blizzards I had ever seen. There were no motorways then, and our difficulties began at Highgate. There was a hold-up of traffic, as vehicles struggled to climb the hill. At first it seemed to be an impasse, when there appeared out of the blue, as it were, gangs of men with lengths of rope, who took charge of the situation. Several men at each end of a rope, would tackle a vehicle in trouble by passing the rope across the back. Then on either side of the motor, they pulled it up the hill. This was repeated time and time again. Our turn came quickly, and we were on our way once more. I have not seen this successful manoeuvre repeated since.

The rest of the journey entailed driving cautiously against the blizzard. Eventually we arrived at the entrance to the farm, a gated road, and perforce finished the journey to the caravan on foot. Wearied as we were, the warmth of the caravan, hot drinks and the meal which Rennie had prepared, were an ideal recompense for our travail. Later, with an effort, I made my way back along the gated road, to see to the car for the night. The snow had increased to such an extent, that I could not find it.

Next morning a snowplough cleared a passage along the road, but unfortunately buried my car under a wall of snow about 20 foot deep. It vas not seen again until the thaw in late April. Next morning I had my clinics to attend. I telephoned from the farm to say I might be late, and set off on foot for the main road. To my relief this had been kept clear by the use of salt and snowploughing.

With relief, I boarded a bus for Leicester. This became my regular daily habit until after the final thaw in early May.

The village of Thurlaston was cut off for several days, and began to run out of essential supplies. The most pressing needs were petrol and bread. In the caravan we needed both, and when in Leicester, I tried to find a sledge, there was not one to be had, so I decided to make one.

I went to the woodyard, only to discover that the firm was forbidden to sell any wood, as it was all required to make things for export. Eventually, I was allowed to buy some poor quality off-cuts of wood. Fortunately, nails and screws were not restricted, and eventually I knocked up a sledge of sorts. I loaded it with a 5 gallon drum of paraffin, a number of loaves, and other things we were short of.

It would have taken several hours to trudge through the snow from Leicester to Thurlaston, but I managed to get permission to load the packed sledge onto a bus. At the turning for our village, I got off the bus and started towing the sledge. I had telephoned the farm, and Mr. Benbow, the farmer, had told Rennie I was on my way. She kept an eye out for my arrival. As soon as she saw me in the distance, she left the caravan and set out to meet me. It was only possible to travel on foot along the tops of the hedges. When we were close enough to wave and call to each other, Rennie suddenly disappeared from view. She had slipped off the hedge. We were laughing so much as I joined her, that it took some time for us both to scramble back to the safety of the hedge-top. Rennie had had no idea that she was walking on top of the hedge, for it looked like an ordinary path of beaten snow. We scrambled to the caravan, unloaded the sledge and enjoyed our tea with Morris, who had remained ignorant of his Mother's disappearing act.

Benbow, the farmer, and Morris were great pals. Morris loved to accompany him around the farm. Benbow used his tractor, with a large sheet of galvanised iron as a trailer. One day the tractor with trailer passed us as we were walking along. There was Morris standing on the trailer, with a staff in his hand. As they turned away from us, Morris, waving his staff, shouted, "Farewell England!" He was about five then.

The farmer had a remarkable horse, very canny in fact. It was almost impossible to stop him from straying, if that was his whim. This clever beast had found out how to open gates, He would release latches, draw bolts, and undo hitches. Unfortunately he omitted to close the gates behind him. He was a favourite, but his wanderlust had to be checked, and finally padlocks defeated even his ingenuity!

In the meantime, I had been to an estate agent to enquire about a house. No suitable accommodation was available until June when, at last, a house, with a large garden sloping down to the river Soar, came on the market. It was a 'one carriage' house with a stable, carriage house (an excellent garage), and front garden. Rennie and I did not hesitate to secure it. By now my car had been found, cleaned, and reconditioned.

****

What furniture we had in store was brought to Leicester and installed. The windows were long and the problem of how to provide enough material for Rennie to make curtains, at first seemed baffling. All curtain materials had been bought up since the war ended. At last this difficulty was solved by an enterprising individual, who bought up quantities of sailcloth. This was very heavy canvas, originally made for the old time sailing ships, such as the "Cutty Sark." He had the lengths dyed attractive colours and advertised them. The weight of the canvas was such that a sail-maker's palm was almost needed to finish the curtains. Rennie stuck at it, however, and eventually she had the satisfaction of seeing her storm canvas curtains with pelmets, admired by all.

My out-patient clinics and operating sessions kept me hard at work. A special children's small hospital had been set up, to deal with the huge waiting list of children with chronically infected tonsils, and middle ear disease. The unit had three wards with ten beds in each. This enabled ten children to be admitted to each ward in sequence, with two days convalescence. I also had similar sessions at Markfield, Hinckley, and Market Bosworth. This period was before antibiotics were generally available.

Today, it is often claimed that many children had their tonsils removed needlessly, but without the revolution brought about by the advent of antibiotics, many of them would have succumbed to related diseases such as bronchitis, pneumonia, otitis media, or rheumatic fever, to mention some of the sequelae of chronic upper respiratory infections of childhood.

Waring and I decided to build a small boat, as the river flowed at the bottom of our garden. We were still up against the difficulty of buying wood, and so we had to make do with anything available. Collecting together branches of fir trees, in the garden, for ribs, the old draining board in the kitchen, some old battens, a tarpaulin and a gallon of tar, with galvanised nails and some screws, we started building the hull of the 'Goblin'. Rennie made a set of sails, and with a mast securely stepped, we had an efficient small sailing skiff. A pair of rowlocks and oars completed the nautical outfit. Every member of the family enjoyed trips in the 'Goblin', needless to say not all at the same time. Two adults of average weight was the limit, perhaps with Pedro, the terrier.

On one occasion the weight was ignored with fortunately no untoward result. We had taken the 'Goblin' to the Trent.

The river was wider than the Soar, and there was a ferryman, who took passengers across for a few pence. He was not on duty one day when Morris, who was now quite an expert oarsman, was in the 'Goblin' on his own at the water's edge, when a giant of a man asked him to take him across the river but this huge fellow called another heavyweight to join him. When these two massive individuals got into the skiff, she was down to almost water-level. The freeboard was little more than an inch. Meanwhile, the rest of us were expecting Morris to join us for our picnic tea, when, to our alarm suddenly we saw Morris rowing the grossly overladen Goblin across the river.

I rushed down to try to stop such a risky trip. Alas, too late.

Hurriedly I looked around for a boat, if a rescue were needed. However, by the time I had the attention of a man with a boat, the Goblin had made a safe passage. I watched, as two obviously frightened passengers landed safely. From their appearance, at that distance, they had been scared to the limit in midstream. As they reached terra firma on the far bank, they scrambled out and almost fled, with no word of thanks for Morris.

He rowed back with the Goblin practically prancing, now freed from its cumbrous cargo. On joining us, he appeared quite unconscious of the risk he had run, and was surprised at our anxiety. We warned him of the danger of overloading the Goblin, and told him to ask permission from us, before acting as ferryman in future. Then we all tucked into our picnic tea.

The registration number of the Humber Snipe was BAA BAA 414. We were going on holiday one year, towing our caravan, and caught up with a similar outfit which was travelling slowly, their registration number was DOG DOG *****. As we overtook them, our four children shouted out "WOOF WOOF WOOF!" but they soon accelerated, and their children retaliated by yelling "BAA, BAA, BAA, BAA!!"

Later we found ourselves neighbours in a campsite.

What pleasure comes from such encounters on holiday! Our riverside house had its disadvantages. It was near the gasworks and, with the breeze in the right (or wrong?) direction, we were in an atmosphere reminiscent of rotten eggs. This was only occasionally, but the chance of buying a thatched 'Cruck' cottage in the village of Billesdon was irresistible.

Such a move would have one advantage, it was eight to nine miles on the road to Oundle, and Waring would be starting there in the near future. We had been in our riverside home for just about two years, and there was no difficulty in finding a buyer. The disadvantage would be the increased mileage to and from Leicester and my outlying clinics.

The cottage was in the process of being re-thatched and modernised, and would be ready for us in a few months. Rennie was in her element making new curtains, and she spent hours making carpeting. She made hundreds of square feet, working in our caravan with a special pedal attachment. A truly remarkable achievement. Some of the carpet is still in use today. There was a much larger garden, a good garage, and of course all modern conveniences.

Almost as soon as we moved, we were in trouble. Our terrier was unused to sheep, he started to 'run them'. Two had to be killed and after compensating the farmer, we were told there was no cure, and that Toby would have to be put down. We were most distressed about this, when another farmer called to see us and was convinced he could cure Toby. We jumped at this prospect, and witnessed the cure of sheep worrying. We took Toby to his farm. The farmer opened the gate to a small yard and said, "Let the dog in." We let Toby in and when he saw a ram, he charged at him, but to Toby's surprise, the ram butted him, and then chased him around the yard, butting him again and again. A chastened Toby was eventually let out, and he never chased another sheep. His lesson was truly learnt.

1949 was the appointed year for the change-over from a Voluntary Hospital Service, and the Local Authority Hospitals and Clinics, to the National Health Service, with the start of a State General Practice Service. All doctors were assured that they would be no worse off.

After the change-over my duties were altered, and I was told to take over operating sessions at Oakham or Uppingham. I forget which it was where I attended for my first session, but I found myself in a tense atmosphere of suspicious antagonism. Towering in the centre of the hospital staff was the indignant figure of an elderly surgeon. He hailed me with the belligerent announcement, "I am the

Ear, Nose and Throat Surgeon to this hospital, and have been for the past twenty years. I have sent away all cases for operation today, as I do not recognise you as being on this hospital's staff!"

Then I understood the dilemma Toby had been in, when confronted by the ram.

(Through my mind flashed the quotation "But me no buts"). However I answered, as reasonably as I could, "I regret the session had to be cancelled, this must have been distressing for patients and relatives. I suggest that over a cup of coffee, we can discuss how this unfortunate episode could have occurred."

It turned out to be due to confusion somewhere among the higher echelons of the management staff of the embryo National Health Service. We enjoyed our cup of coffee, and when I left the atmosphere was almost one of cordiality.

Obviously the error was quite unintentional, and my new appointment was at a different hospital.

Somewhat unexpectedly, we discovered that thatched roofs had some peculiar disadvantages. The thatching was secured in place with galvanised iron wire netting. One morning I was wakened by a crescendo of twitterings, which seemed to increase to an agonising intensity. Almost panic stricken myself at this so close and intolerable commotion, I hurried down to see what was happening. To my amazement one section of the thatch was covered by crowd of agitated sparrows. They flew off, it seemed to me with reluctance, as I approached, and there was revealed a pending avian tragedy. A sparrow had somehow got under the wire net, and was helplessly trapped.

What amazed me was the concern, and frantic efforts of a whole flock to succour a member in distress.

I felt I must try to free the captive, and decided to cut some of the wire netting, so as to give room for the bird to escape, I failed, because as soon as the pressure on the sparrow eased it dragged itself into a more hopeless position, and eventually choked itself. The flock stayed nearby, silent now, and it seemed to me, almost cognisant of the attempted rescue.

On another occasion, the thatch caused us anxiety when it was invaded by mice. From the amount of debris which issued from their lairs, we feared, that unless some effective way was to be found of getting rid of them, our thatch would be destroyed. I was getting anxious, and wondered if the insurance might cover re-thatching.

I mentioned this to a villager, adding that I wondered what the legal position was. He went straight to the previous owner and told him I was taking legal action against him!

Having explained that misunderstanding away, I was feeling chary, when another local householder mentioned that he could tell me how to get rid of the mice. I doubted the efficacy of his cure, but I was quite wrong, for it proved a winner. His instructions I followed in detail. He advised "Back your car as near the affected area of thatch as you can. Fit a hose over the exhaust pipe, and push the other end of the hose well into the thatch. Start the engine and leave it running for an hour or two." It worked for there was no further trouble from mice. What happened to them is a mystery, but I hope they left for adventures elsewhere.

The cottage was near the church and vicarage. We were members of the congregation, and the Vicar and his wife and daughter were on friendly terms.

Rennie was, and is, a communicant, but I have never been a confirmed member of the church, as I cannot bring myself to accept the wording of the Athanasian Creed.

I was therefore surprised to be asked to read the first lesson at Sunday morning service. I forget which it was, but I remember recalling the words of one of the Hebrew prophets. Finding myself at the lectern, conscious of the solemnity of the occasion, and knowing that Christians had worshipped for generations under this roof, I became overawed. It seemed to me, the prophet himself was influencing my voice as I read.

****

I noticed Paddy praying, later I asked her about her prayer.

She was embarrassed, but finally told me, that she prayed,

"Dear God, please stop Father."

My utterances had been bordering on the melodramatic. This reminded me of the advice of the Medical Council: "Never become personally or emotionally involved!" All the same, I feel the prophet may well have been. Paddy's remark also reminded me of the first melodrama I saw when a boy. It was at the Theatre Royal, in High Street, Peckham. In the grand finale, the wealthy villain having failed to ruin the heroine, had a heart attack, and perished on the centre of the stage.

Then stepping to the front centre, a clergyman actor raised his arms to heaven, and cried in a loud voice,

"Of what avail are all his millions now!" CURTAIN.

I trust my reading fell far short of that.

Rennie and I had hoped that Paddy would take up art, but she elected to do drama. (This was before my reading in church). An appointment was made for me to attend at R.A.D.A. on her behalf. I duly did so, and the greeting I received was fulsome but alas there was no place for her at that time. This was a a similar circumstance as befell her sister's application to study medicine.

However, a place was available at the Birmingham School of Dramatic Art and Speech Training. There Paddy qualified L.R.A.M. in Speech and Drama.

Among the ruins of Coventry Cathedral the school performed a final play, which was a soul searching production of The Trial of Christ.

Paddy married one of her fellow graduates, who later left this country for a career in the United States. Paddy soon joined him, but the marriage was not a happy one.

Since then Paddy has prospered in the States, and has now retired, and begun to develop her talents in the art world. We have received some charming gifts from her, especially in 'stained glass'.

Elizabeth had finished her training as a radiographer. She applied once more to start training in medicine, but was advised to continue in radiography, as there was still a long queue for medicine. She applied successfully for the post of radiographer to the General Hospital in Guernsey, Channel Isles. Later she married a Guernsey artist, Kenneth Hill. He bought a piece of ground near the shore, and built a marvellous family house. They now have four children, and three grandchildren. Needless to say, Elizabeth has retired from radiography.

Waring started at Oundle School and enjoyed life there, especially woodworking and cricket.

Morris was still at preparatory school, and was due to start as a boarder at a Woodard School at Bloxham.

The years were passing, and 1951 was the year of the Festival of Britain. This was celebrated with the building of the National Theatre and other halls of entertainment on South Bank.

I recall one particular very impressive attraction. It was a model history of mankind, showing the development of homo-sapiens. The small figures were exquisitely made, and I feel it is such a loss that they have not been retained on South Bank. The Festival was celebrated throughout the land, including Billesdon.

Paddy was made one of the organisers of the revelery, which embraced fancy dress. There were many old time characters: Dicken's Mr. Pickwick arriving in a stage coach was to open the proceedings! A drunken villager would sell his wife. There was to be a runaway marriage of the squire's daughter, the couple being pursued by the irate father.

With the old stage coach available, Rennie suggested to the vicar, whose eyes twinkled at the thought, that Dick Turpin should hold up the coach in approved dramatic style, demanding "Your money or your life"!

To my surprise, I was picked on to play the drunk who sold his wife. But at a rehearsal, spectators objected to my performance thinking I was genuinely 'one over the eight'. So I became the irate father instead, and at the reconciliation, I took advantage of the opportunity to 'Kiss the bride'. Much to her surprise!

About this time changes were afoot in the Health Service, which consisted of reorganising and regrading the medical staff. This was a long affair, and was carried out by a committee of the old voluntary staff and ministry officials.

Two grades of specialists were to be formed:- Consultants and Senior Hospital Medical Officers.

Eventually, this would have unexpected results, and cause great consternation among specialists, but not for some time.

Meanwhile all the nation was looking forward to the Coronation in 1953. Life was full of changes, one of which was the building of motorways. The M1 was to be the first, and would make the journey from Leicester to London so much easier. During its construction, Rennie and I were travelling back to Billesden, when we pulled off with the caravan in a quiet lay-by for the night.

This was before the numerous camping sites that have sprung up since were available. Little did we know what awaited us early next morning. It was well after midnight when we finally snuggled down after an enjoyable supper.

What we had not realised was that on the other side of the hedge a by-pass for the Ml/Al was being made. About 4 a.m. mechanical earth diggers and removal lorries arrived with concrete mixers, and judging by their voices, most enthusiastic motorway builders. The noises were so loud, penetrating and at all levels so extreme, we decided to make ourselves scarce, without our usual 'getting up' procedure. We soon found another lay-by, where we rested, and finished getting up. Then we had breakfast, and the fact that it was a lovely day, and that bird song replaced the racket of man's activities, we more than cheered up.

One day, whilst operating in Leicester, Rennie rang me up with the sad news of the tragic death of her brother-in-law, Sidney, Eva's husband, as he was singing in the church choir.

Eva was prostrated with grief. Rennie and all the family did what they could to support her during her anguish. Her three daughters, bereft of their loving father, were overwhelmed, and suffered piteously. Rennie's compassion and help must have meant a great deal to her sister and nieces during the weeks following Sidney's death.

Life, however, has to continue for the bereaved as well as for others.

A short time afterwards, I had a telephone call from the Sister-in-charge of a Home for Educationally Subnormal Children - Would the Ear, Nose and Throat surgeon please call to see her about some of the children?

When I did call, she explained her problems. A number of the children suffered from frequent bouts of tonsillitis, others with a nasal discharge, and some with recurrent discharge from their ears - Would I examine them, and see her with regard to treatment for them?

This I duly did and reported that there were a number of cases of chronic tonsillitis with frequent recurrent acute exacerbations. Other children had enlarged adenoids, causing nasal obstruction and postnasal discharge, with the danger of bronchitis or pneumonia, and sometimes leading to infection of the ears, both acute and chronic, with possible subsequent deafness.

Sister had expected this report, and realised that there could be no improvement in the general health of the community, unless the sources of re-infection were treated by appropriate surgery.

She explained the difficulty regarding surgical treatment.

The children needing operation were supposed to be admitted to the Royal Infirmary for treatment. Unfortunately trouble arose because the children were taken from their normal surroundings and cared for by strangers. This was a terrifying experience for subnormal children, and created a most unhappy atmosphere in the ward for the other children. The tendency to procrastinate was unavoidable. Had I any suggestion? I replied that an unofficial committee of three:- Sister, the anaesthetist, Dr. McNeil, (she was a children's anaesthetist par excellence), and I, should meet to consider what to do. We did so, and the first question was, was there a treatment room at the home suitable for use as a temporary surgical theatre. There was, and I had my portable operating table.

Could we deal with any possible emergencies however unlikely? Blood grouping of the children was done on those for operation, and liaison was arranged with the pathological department of the Royal infirmary.

The worst cases were selected for the first session and duly operated on one morning. All the children did well. At this stage, the committee of management was informed that the operating session had taken place.

As expected, I was requested to attend the next session of the committee. At the meeting the Chairman asked me - Why was the committee not informed that it was proposed to operate at the home? I replied that "I was sure all members of the committee realised the alarming condition of the affected children, and were aware of the difficulties associated with their admission to hospital."

I thought that individually, each member of the committee would personally approve of my action, but as a committee, they would seek authority from higher up. I accepted full responsibility for the action, which had become so urgent.

Eventually the Chairman thanked me, but requested no such further action should be taken without the committee's approval.

The matter was referred to higher authority, where it was decided that children needing surgical treatment should, in future, be admitted to the Royal Infirmary.

Fortunately, the immediate situation had been remedied, and in a year or so antibiotics were freely available.

Soon, with new antibiotics being discovered, a genuine wonder cure for tuberculosis "streptomycin" was the latest breakthrough. The effect of this antibiotic was amazing, sanatoria became superfluous, and many chest physicians, who specialised in tuberculosis, became either redundant, or had to choose another branch of medicine.

This was at the time of the regrading of medical specialists in the National Health Service.

We had been resident in Billesdon for three years, when the Senior Nose, Ear, and Throat Surgeon at the Leicester Royal Infirmary, sent for me to tell me that, in spite of all he could do, the grading committee had downgraded my appointment from Consultant to Senior Hospital Medical Officer, which affected my personal grading.

****

At first the personal grading did not seem so important, as I have already mentioned that the Minister of Health had stated that no doctors would be suffer financially.

How mistaken I was, for my salary was reduced to less than half.

This placed me in an impossible financial position. To make matters worse I realised that I was badly affected as regarded income tax. This was charged on the average income for the present, and the two preceding years.

I tried to appeal, but there was no such procedure until later. At the grading of posts, all the senior members of the old voluntary hospital staffs were classed as consultants, but most of the senior specialists employed by local authorities were categorised Senior Hospital Medical Officers.

The gross reduction in my finances compelled me to take our son, Waring, away from Oundle school, at that critical point in his education when he was about to take his preliminary examination for entrance to university.

He continued his studies by taking on a correspondence course and working in the caravan. He successfully passed his entrance examination. His next step was to pass his first year's examination before starting his clinical studies at hospital. He had nearly completed it when he was faced with a dramatic (for him) choice. The date of the last minor oral examination clashed with the hospital team's cricket match. Confident that playing for the hospital would offset his non-attendance at the minor oral examination, he played cricket, with the unfortunate consequence that it cost him two marks.

The post-war national service of two years was still operative, and in spite of all I could do by means of interviews and letters (because he was short of those two vital marks), he was called up. He spent the next two years in the R.A.F.

This deferred the date of his final qualifying for that period. For the record, I believe the hospital won that cricket match! To add insult to injury, at a meeting of all area specialists at the Leicester

Royal Infirmary after one or two general matters had been discussed, all S.H.M.O's were asked to leave whilst the Consultants discussed the remaining items on the agenda.

This arrogant demand infuriated all the S.H.M.O's.

On the way out, I asked all the S.H.M.O's to meet in the Staff Room to organise a protest.

Only one S.H.M.O. beside myself stayed behind. The others were too disheartened to do more than grumble, however downcast they felt. We two decided to consider ourselves representatives of all the S.H.M.O's in the Leicester area, who had attended the meeting, we had our session, as representatives of them all. One would propose a motion the other seconded it and it would be passed, not surprisingly, unanimously.

We decided on the following procedures:

1. to ask the B.M.A. for a room for S.H.M.O's to meet
2. as the Consultants Committee of the B.M.A. must have agreed the new gradings, we decided to start organising on our own
3. to circulate the medical staffs of all the major hospitals in the country to the effect that there would be a meeting of S.H.M.O's at B.M.A. Headquarters to discuss the position,

and what action to take.

This involved sending out hundreds of letters.

Paddy, who had not yet gone to the States, was a most valuable help in addressing and posting the correspondence.

The day of the meeting arrived. When I reached the B.M.A. Hdqrs. at Tavistock Square, a committee room had been put at my disposal. As the hour for the meeting approached, so many S.H.M.O's arrived that a much larger room was needed. The numbers increased so rapidly that finally the Great Hall had to be used, even then some S.H.M.O's had to stand. To give some idea of the problem, the total number of S.H.M.O's was between 2,000 and 3,000. Not all were present of course. I was made Chairman, (I had stuck my neck out), and finally I left the meeting, laden down with subscriptions.

Eventually, over the years, over 2,000 S.H.M.O's were regraded to Consultant.

I was approached early on as to whether, if a select number were upgraded, would I accept that as a settlement? I replied "No." The years were passing, whilst meetings continued with the number of regradings steadily increasing, and my retirement age was approaching.

I had been forced to reduce my cost of living.

The situation was compounded by the fact that my sister-in-law decided to sell her house at Chiselhurst, and Rennie and I were prepared to share a house in Leicester with her, if we could locate a suitable one.

As a result of the drop in income, our lovely thatched cottage had to be sold and cheaper accommodation found.

Waring had to be taken away from Oundle at the end of the year. I used a motor bicycle instead of a car.

The cottage fetched a good price and I bought a semi-detached four storey house in Leicester.

Some alterations had to be made to cater for Eva and her two daughters. Everything seemed to revolve around a door, which had to be hung in a different position. This I decided to do myself, but I found that part of the operation involved my standing upside down.

I managed successfully, and then ran downstairs to put the tools back in the workshop. Arriving in the garden I promptly 'blacked out'. I 'came to' to find Pedro, our new terrier, vigorously licking my face! The look of relief on his face was followed by leaps and bounds plus tail wagging.

He was an exceptionally intelligent animal. As a puppy, I noticed he made an almost human vocal sound when he yawned. By applauding this, I gradually encouraged him to utter a distinct "Halloo." He used this to good purpose for he developed a daily round of the neighbours. He would wack at a door with his tail, and when it was opened, he adopted a begging stance, and uttered his "Halloo." It was no wonder that he put on too much weight!

Private operating in Leicester was limited, as there were only a few private beds, and these were booked ahead by consultants, with one exception, not one would book for Friday the 13th. They were not in the least superstitious, but they preferred to play safe! So, every Friday the 13th I did my private operating. I was appointed as a Consultant Specialist to the Ministry of Pensions. This meant weekly journeys to London. Unfortunately the railway system was in a bad state after the war, and trains were often late, so I had to give the pension work up. The final train journey I made was with a new Diesel locomotive, supposed "pride of the line." Regrettably it broke down, and was towed to London by an old steamer. Luckily the train arrived in London just in time for me to catch my return to Leicester.

As chairman of the S.H.M.O. Group of the B.M.A., I had unwittingly taken on almost a full time job. I was determined not to let the campaign flag, and started a monthly S.H.M.O. Bulletin for distribution among all members. Regional meetings were held at least six monthly. The case for the Group was pushed at each annual meeting of the B.M.A. for five years. Opposition from the Ministry and the higher Consultant ranks was vigorous. Eventually after my retirement in 1965, I continued the struggle, and the S.H.M.O, grade was finally abolished.

When I retired, the British Medical Association gave a farewell luncheon. I was presented by the B.M.A. with a personal portrait, which was exhibited at the Royal Academy Exhibition the same year. Elizabeth's husband, Kenneth Hill, had painted it. To add to my pleasure, the S.H.M.O. Group gave me a handsome cheque in appreciation of my efforts. Rennie was present and she had a husband full of gratitude for the wonderful support she had given through this long and tedious struggle. Life in Leicester had its advantages, as we soon rediscovered. We enjoyed our visits to the theatre, where we saw T.S. Eliot's "Murder in the Cathedral", the poetic drama woven around the death of Thomas à Becket.

The repertory company produced many interesting plays until its untimely end from lack of support.

Today, we see some members of the repertory company on television, especially one of the knights who acted on King Henry's cry "Will no one rid me of this turbulent priest!"

At the side of our new house, a deep cutting had been made for access to a small nursery, which was now used as allotments for local residents. It contained a large greenhouse, which had been built probably in the Victorian era. This we rented for a small sum. It was heated by means of a coal fire, which we rarely used. It was large enough to produce peaches, grapes, tomatoes, lettuces and early seedlings for planting out.

There was room beside it for our caravan to stand. At the end of our garden, there was a private drive from a side road, which gave access to our garage and those of neighbours.

It was badly maintained, and became muddy, with potholes filled with water whenever it rained. One day I noticed that the roof of a neighbouring house was being repaired, and the old earthenware tiles had been dumped into a lorry, ready for removal.

I spotted the lorry driver getting into his seat, and went to ask him "What is going to happen to that load of old tiles?"

"I'm taking it to the dump," he replied.

"Couldn't you dump it here?" I enquired.

He jumped at the idea. "Do you mean that?"

"Yes, I do" I affirmed. Without further ado, he tipped the lorry, spilling the lot. There must have been two tons of broken tiles. The load blocked the lane completely. Hurriedly I fetched my roller, sledge-hammer, spade and barrow. I had about an hour before the return of the first neighbour on his motor-bike. Working flat out, I had just cleared a way, when he arrived. His language was unrepeatable. After he had cooled slightly he demanded to know who was responsible? He would have the law on whoever it was! When calm enough to listen, I explained, "I'm to blame." I couldn't let pass such an opportunity of resurfacing our drive-in with its potholes and mud. It hadn't cost anything other than a little hard work. Just then the next resident, a woman, turned up driving her small car, crunching and rolling on the loose slates. Her language, although much more moderate, was no less irate. They joined forces and condemned me for acting without having a meeting of all residents. They seemed quite oblivious of the fact it would have taken days at least to convene such a meeting, and if the decision had not been made within a few minutes, the chance would have been lost.

It was a Saturday, and I promised that by Monday morning we would have a newly surfaced spick and span gravelled drive. I hinted that I would appreciate any help, but none was forthcoming. True to my prognosis, on the Monday the drive was an example of a nearly perfect gravelled lane, and eventually I was rewarded by the gracious approval of all the users thereof. I soon gave up using a motor-bike, after I met with an unusual occurrence when returning from London. I was in a stream of traffic, mostly heavy lorries, when I noticed danger ahead. The tarpaulin covering the load on a lorry in front, seemed to heave about, and suddenly a large bale of straw dropped down in front of me. It rolled towards me, I could not avoid it and, amid the screeching of brakes from the lorry behind, I crashed into the centre of the mass. Fortunately, the driver had seen what was about to happen for his braking was instantaneous. Both my motor bike and I were entangled within the centre of the bale, while the lorry in front sped blissfully on its way. The driver of the lorry behind me got down, and amid laughter from him, myself and bystanders, my machine and I, a battered looking scarecrow myself, were freed from the now burst bale. I suffered no permanent damage, nor did the bike, and the lorry driver and I bade each other farewell with gratitude on my part, and much amusement on his.

This accident demonstrated to me how helpless one can be on only two wheels, and I have distrusted motor bikes since then.

****

A few years after Eva had been with us at Leicester, she decided to move to Cornwall with her daughter, Janet, to be near Bridget, her eldest daughter and her husband, Dennison. They had a lovely farm bordering on the river Tamar. We spent many enjoyable weekends with them using our caravan. Eva had a small house in Poughill, a village near Bude, and only a few miles from the farm.

It was in 1958 that we were on holiday with Eva, when Rennie and I went for a walk to the nearby beach, Norcot Mouth. On the way down I noticed a field with a 'For Sale' notice on the gate. As we were walking back Rennie suddenly said to me, "If only we could buy a piece of ground here."

"I've seen the very piece," I replied, and forthwith we returned to look at it closely. There was the Atlantic in the background about two miles away. It looked the perfect site for my retirement, which was due in another three years.

The agent was in Bude, so we at once called at his office. I asked the price which the agent said was £350. This was too much for me at that time, but the Agent enquired "Will you make an offer?" I did. "£250," I said.

To my surprise he asked for my cheque which he accepted, and we became the proud owners of about half an acre of Cornwall overlooking the Atlantic ocean.

As now owners, we opened the gate, removed the "For Sale" notice and surveyed our domain of the future. To us it seemed perfect, but we were rather knocked back when a local farmer, who was passing, told us that the council had condemned it.

They had hoped to build an extension of the neighbouring cottages on that piece of ground. However the surveyor had condemned it as waterlogged, therefore unfit for building. Of course it was high summer when we first saw the field. Apparently it had proved useless for growing crops. Now we knew why the price was so reasonable.

Would it be possible to drain the piece of ground? Closer

examination revealed two ditches. One at the side, bordering the council cottages, and the other along the south side, facing the sea. The council had not attempted to drain the land on account of the cost. No longer downhearted, Rennie and I decided to find out if we could drain it ourselves. We were not rushed for time. First the ditch on the seaward side would have to be cleared, then the whole area drained by land drainage pipes. This involved cutting channels from the roadway to the far ditch.

After I had cleared the ditch, Rennie and I laid in the channels, about 600 clay pipes, each approximately 18 inches long with a small gap between them. They were then covered with soil. When it rained, we had the childish excitement of seeing the surface water pouring from our channels into the ditch. Our future home we ordered from Guildway, who supplied a sectional cedar wood bungalow, and recommended a builder to lay the foundations and main drainage. We insisted on floor heating, which was put in with the foundation.

The bungalow arrived on two huge lorries, and for the next couple of years, during holidays, our two sons erected the building, and tiled the roof. Not without some difficulty when some of the roof trusses slipped, and grazed Morris's head. Building over a long period of time had its difficulties. The first winter, when the bungalow was just a shell, the supporting partitions had not yet been erected; when there was the worst gale for many years, it blew with its full force straight from the Atlantic over the bungalow, which was distorted and left leaning precariously inland. Hurriedly summoned, our builder produced steel hawsers and, with them securely anchored, gradually winched the structure upright. Once the internal walls were finished, there was no danger of a recurrence.

In another six months, we were able to spend our holidays in our seaside home. There was a great deal to be done before I finally retired.

Rennie was busy making curtains once more, and helping me to cover the concrete floors with parquet flooring, (no old engine oil and paraffin on this occasion). I dread to think what might have happened with floor heating.

1961 was the year of my retirement from the Health Service, for I would be 65 years of age in September. Our prospects could not have been better. With the generous cheque from the S.H.M.O. Group, and the maturity of my life insurance, we were at last free from financial anxiety.

Elizabeth was happily married in Guernsey. She and Kenneth had two children, Suzanne and William. Rennie and I were proud grandparents. Paddy had left to join her husband in New York.

Unfortunately disaster struck at home. The cutting to the nursery at the side of our house had to some extent weakened the foundations on that side, this coupled with the very dry spell, and shrinkage of the clay substratum, caused the outside wall of the building to collapse. About one third of the house was affected and a demolition firm had to be sent for in an effort to save the remaining structure. In its present state the property was valueless, and I was faced with demolition costs, apart from repairs, if they were possible.

There could be no truer parallel than that between ourselves and Humpty-Dumpty of the nursery rhyme - "Who had a great fall, and all the King's horses and all the King's men couldn't put Humpty together again."

Our house on a wall had a great fall, and the law and insurance couldn't put our house together again.

The law said our house was now a dangerous structure, and we were responsible for either making it safe, or for its demolition.

The insurance policy did not cover weakening of the foundation, or the shrinkage of the substratum.

However, the insurance company pointed out that a few years back there had been a mild earthquake in the area. If the surveyor agreed that the earth tremor might have been partly to blame, they would consider making an 'ex gratia' contribution to the costs.

To our chagrin and intense disappointment the surveyor flatly refused.

We had various estimates made of the cost of demolition of the house, possible part demolition and repair of the remaining structure. The first would leave only a site, and the cost would been such that we would be left almost destitute. The second was a possibility. On consulting a builder, he said this was feasible, if he could have used the old bricks. New ones would increase the cost beyond our limit, having the old ones cleaned would be just as expensive.

Rennie came to the rescue: "Why cannot we clean them ourselves?" There were thousands of them lying in the cutting. Together we tackled the job. I say we, but I was away working at hospitals all day, and could only help part time.

Rennie wore thick rubber gloves, and with a builder's trowel she cleaned brick after brick, and the heap of old mortar chippings increased hourly. We were recommended a builder, who was a Cornishman, his name was Pengelly. His enthusiasm and energy put new life into us. Gradually, the new, though reduced in size, house arose. When completed, there remained the interior rooms to construct. Waring stepped in at this stage and accomplished that task, just before the local authority brought in certain specifications, which would have considerably increased the cost. The house was now in a sound condition and fit to live in and I decided to tidy up the cutting, and started to remove some of the heap of mortar debris, when I noticed some greenish buds. Working cautiously, to my surprise I uncovered some of the most appetising stalks of rhubarb I had ever seen.

Our move to our Cornish retirement home was drawing near.

There were retirement parties at hospitals and clinics. Gifts included a handsome set of glass tumblers and flagon, a solid silver coffee set, a garden settee and chairs, and stainless steel garden tools.

The Leicester house was sold for a reasonable sum, and although our capital had been reduced to a fraction of its original value, it was with high hopes and much joy that we left Leicester and set forth for our retirement in North Cornwall. It was now late autumn, but Moorcroft, our new home, looked warmly welcoming amid the autumn colours, with the vivid blue of the Atlantic background. Rennie and I will always cherish the memory of that day.

We arrived with the van bringing our furniture. It all fitted in place, just as we had hoped. Our fears that, as much of it consisted of antiques, it would look out of place, proved to be groundless. In fact when my sister-in-law, Eva, first saw our new home complete with Rennie's curtains, she exclaimed "Quite charming, quite charming." Eva was of a critical disposition and her approval was praise indeed.

The main water supply ended at the council cottages, and a temporary hose was connected to the council main which reached Moorcroft by way of a meadow and over a hedge. This was of great interest to the cows, who grazed in the field. They licked it assiduously, as though they were bovine water diviners. The kitchen was a joy for Rennie and there was an excellent larder. This is a feature often absent in these days of freezers and refrigerators.

****

The large garden, which surrounded the house, was my main consideration. I tackled it in ignorance and indeed recklessly. I ordered the smallest 'commercial' greenhouse, and then from a nursery in South Devon I ordered 200 young apple trees as well as various fruit bushes.

Then I learnt, that owing to the heavy deposits of salt from the sea with inland breees, apples would not thrive. I next sought advice from the Agricultural Department of Exeter. To my surprise, I had a letter from the head, saying how delighted he was at hearing from me. He suggested a day when he could call and advise. I was astonished at this enthusiastic response, and on the appointed day I waited with unusual interest for his arrival. He came by car, and I was outside to welcome him. When he got out of the car, and I introduced myself, he looked startled, and asked "You are not G.W.Robinson?"

"Indeed I am" I replied.

His next remark was "I heard you were dead, I mean the Robinson I knew." This put me in a state of confusion. I wondered briefly, who I really was !

However, we both soon recovered from our uncertainty, and he was anxious to see what should be done to help.

After a quick look around he returned to his car and produced a number of small plastic bags and also a peculiar long sharp stainless shovel. Systematically, he went over the whole of our plot, taking samples of soil and carefully numbering each one. He then said how pleased he was to have met us, would not stop even for a cup of coffee, and drove off with a wave and promise that we should soon hear from him.

The report soon came with detailed recommendations of what should be done, if our apple trees were to have any chance of survival.

The soil was intensely alkaline, we would have to excavate a cubic yard of soil for each tree, and replace it with a compound of peat and soil compost. This meant digging out 60 cubic yards, one for each apple tree. Such a task seemed hopeless, but it was surprising, when Rennie and I set to work, how soon those pits were ready for planting, We had a a small trailer so were able to fetch peat straight from its source at Sedgemoor. Compost we made in quantity, using kitchen waste, and seaweed. which we collected in five gallon drums, brought back and washed repeatedly with rainwater to rid it of sea salt. Fortunately we managed to get a lot done by the end of the year.

The start of 1962 heralded an exceptionally bitter spell of weather for Cornwall. The hose carrying our water froze, once or twice it was possible to thaw it with hot clothes, but this led to a cow chewing it, with predictable failure of our water supply. Luckily, we had collected gallons of rainwater in drums. Boiling this, we managed until the frosts ceased, and our house hose was repaired, this time lagged with cloth. My monthly pension from the Health Service was a poor return for the years of work. I asked the B.M.A. about this and they pointed out that the years spent in the Voluntary Hospital Service did not count. However, they acted on behalf of all doctors in the same plight, and so war service was accepted as counting towards pensions. This helped considerably.

My first cousin, May, whom I described early in my memoirs, was now a widow and, so sad to tell, had lost her only son, who was Padre on the ill-fated "Hood" in 1941. She came to stay with us at Moorcroft for a time. Unfortunately the sight of the sea brought back such bitter memories, that she had to leave and went to a home for the elderly. She died soon afterwards, I shall always remember her with affection.

Our financial situation had greatly improved through locums, and selling apples to the local nursery. They were George Cave, an early variety, ready in July and August; Russets, and Mutsu; a late variety for winter.

The second spring came in and the bluebells were blooming in our garden. This reminded us of the bluebell paradise near Mortenhampstead, which had so entranced us. We decided to take the day off to see once again that lovely feast of colour. When we got to the turning off the main road, at first I thought that I had mistaken it, as it was now larger. When we turned towards the bridge over the brook, we were horrified to see a modern hotel. The meadow was bereft of bluebells, except for one or two bedraggled plants, which had survived in odd corners. There was no shimmer of blue in the sparse wooded slope through which we had emerged so thrilled a few years ago. This experience somehow made us realise that we now faced the future, that the past had irretrievably gone. There are no colour photographs to help recall the beauty of the scene, for that advance in photography was yet to come. We returned, saddened at the loss of so heavenly a vista.

I considered doing consultant work. Up to the age of 72, I did locum consultant jobs in Cornwall, Northern Ireland, and Wales. Some lasted for six months, when Rennie would join me. My six months stint in Ulster was before the present 'troubles' started. The Welsh locum was when the Severn bridge was being built. At that time, there were three ways to Wales, one by road through Gloucester, another by train through the tunnel, and the third by ferry. Our favourite was by ferry, when we could watch the bridge being assembled. We could see huge hollow floating sections of the structure. Each section was towed to its position at water level and then winced into its final location. When finished, it was for a short time I believe the longest suspension bridge in the world.

I had always tried to be careful what I told patients after or during examinations. However I was guilty of once alarming a patient completely unintentionally.

This was a young housewife, who unfortunately was hit by a reversing bus. The impact was on her face. Her nose had been pushed sideways, and flattened against her right cheek. This had happened some weeks before I saw her. On examination the dislocation was severe. If I were to operate, the final cosmetic result was all important. This took time to evaluate.

The patient enquired in anxious tones, "You look worried, Doctor, is it serious?"

Unthinkingly, I replied, "Yes, I am worried it is about asymmetry." I got no further, for she nearly fainted. When she had pulled herself together, she said breathlessly, "You mean it will be fatal?"

"Of course not, whatever gave you that idea?" I responded.

"But you said a cemetery!" she exclaimed. I have been doubly careful since then, not to convey a wrong impression. The final outcome was satisfactory, for when I had freed and removed a fractured bone at the base of the nasal septum, the major section was released and returned almost to normal with an acceptable result.

I did several locums at Truro, and the specialist for whom I was acting had quite a long out-patient waiting list for minor local operations. The out-patient sister kept on producing patients from the waiting list. I found these sessions quite exhausting, and wondered how the consultant had managed to keep going. On one occasion I had to call a halt and rest, while a cup of coffee was brought for me.

Apparently Sister was anxious to reduce the waiting list, and as I was able to treat the patients speedily, she increased the load each session. I was glad when this locum came to its conclusion.

On his return, the consultant demanded in surprise "What has happened to my waiting list?"

I had been used to the old Voluntary Hospital days, when no one thought of leaving until every patient had been seen. When the Regional Hospital Board realised I was 72, the consultant locum tenens posts for me ended, as 70 was the official age limit. I was still able to do general practice locums however.

That same spring there soon followed a stormy few days. Rennie and I drove down to the beach, to collect a further supply of seaweed for compost. The weather was still chilly, so we dressed accordingly in our winter gardening clothes, and ancient wellingtons. We had filled several drums and were carrying them back to the car, when we passed some hardy visitors. Rennie overheard one of them say, "Poor things, they eat that!" We have had many a laugh about that since, yet in a way they may unwittingly have been right. As excellent compost for future crops, we might eventually have done just that.

Poughill Church was at the end of our lane. It had some remarkable wall paintings. They had been covered up during the Cromwellian period, and rediscovered later. One showed Saint Christopher carrying wayfarers across a river.

In the churchyard was interred the skeleton of a prehistoric man, whose remains were revealed after a cliff fall years ago. I have sometimes wondered what rites were performed at the second burial.

We enjoyed the services on Sundays. One Christmas Eve all the pews were illuminated with lighted candles for a carol service. Unfortunately, so much oxygen was sapped from the air by their combustion, that we all felt faint, the candles had to be hurriedly snuffed, and the church doors opened for circulation of fresh air. I have often felt that imitation of candlelight by small electric bulbs was a poor substitute for the flickering flames of the real thing. This experience certainly demonstrated the pros and cons of old ways and the new.

One year, the arrival of spring awoke in us the wanderlust, which had laid dormant for so long.

Rennie and I decided to take the caravan and have a long weekend in Paris. The weather promised to remain fine as we caught the ferry and enjoyed the drive to the Bois de Boulogne. There we found a nice site in the excellent camp. Next morning we decided to walk over the Pont Neuf along the Champs Elysees, to see this lovely city as pedestrians. As we reached the Champs Elysees, the sky clouded over and with the threat of a thunderous downpour, we decided to shelter in an estaminet and enjoy a cup of coffee. There was an inviting vacant table, so we sat down. As we did so, we could not fail to notice an altercation going on between another elderly couple and a worried waiter. We heard him say, "Alors, I fetch Monsieur le Patron," and he disappeared inside. The couple glancing at each other, rose and slipped discreetly away. It was now raining hard. We began to wonder how long we would have to wait before giving our order. Not that it worried us as we were sheltered from the storm.

It was then that Monsieur Le Patron arrived on the scene. He had a ferocious expression, as he glanced around. He spotted us, and approaching our table, he said angrily, "It is not allowed to sit here without ordering something to eat or drink." At this the waiter returned and exclaimed in alarm, "That is not the couple, they have gone."

Monsieur le Patron's expression changed from tigerish anger to one of beatific benevolence, followed by a glowing beam of welcome.

"A thousand apologies Monsieur et Madame. Pierre!" he shouted, and as Pierre rushed to take our order, Monsieur Le Patron withdrew. He reappeared, as Pierre brought our refreshments. Monsieur le Patron placed on the table a vase of flowers, and turning towards Rennie, with the flourish of a courtier, he bowed, pursed his lips, and blew a kiss with his fingers towards the bouquet, and announced "Mais c'est pour vous, Madame."

This episode was the highlight of our weekend, and we returned more than pleased with our Parisian interlude.

Paddy had prospered in San Francisco, and at last was able to buy her own house. This was just outside the 'fault', and so most unlikely to suffer severely during an earthquake. Of course we hoped that one day we should be able to afford the luxury of visiting her.

We had our small annexe, which was complete with kitchen, bathroom and all modern conveniences, and in addition our caravan. I wrote to an agent, who advertised holiday homes. Rather to my surprise the firm sent down a representative to report on the possibilities. His report was favourable, and indeed quite enthusiastic. That summer, we had our first paying guests. One day, they did not return and we worried ourselves stiff. Could they have had an accident? The next morning they were still absent, and we debated as to what we should do. Whether to inform the police. But just as were about to do something, our missing guests turned up, full of their trip to St. Mary's, of the Isles of Scilly.

Later, we mentioned how worried we had been at their absence. We explained that they were our first paying guests and we were novices as far as letting was concerned. They were amused at this, and told us they were honoured at our solicitude for their welfare. They enjoyed their holiday and left, we hope with happy memories.

We saw in the local paper that Penfound Manor, a very old house near Bude, was open to the public on certain days. We decided to visit it. We were more than surprised at the interesting and educational way in which history was displayed, bringing the past vividly to life. We were ushered into the Hall, which had a minstrel gallery at one end. There was a door leading to the kitchen. This was huge with many mediaeval appurtenances still to be seen. There was an open fireplace with a spit, and some old firearms. The kitchen did not open directly to the Hall, for there was a short passageway from the one to the other, with an exceptional feature. There was a brook of clear fresh water flowing over a sandy bottom, from one side to the other. We were told that the servants carrying meals from the rush-strewn kitchen floor to the hall, walked with bare feet through the current of clear water, which crossed the passage, and thus arrived to serve meals for Master, Mistress, and all the company with clean feet. However true that may have been, Rennie and I were able to verify another remarkable piece of history.

On the first floor, as we were ushered into the main bedroom, I could hardly believe what I saw. There before me, was the identical double bed from Hall Place, Bexley. It was the same one from a galleon of the Spanish Armada, which was wrecked off the Cornish coast. I cannot vouch for the accuracy of the story how the bed came back to Cornwall.

When the Countess of Limerick died, Hall Place was taken over by the Council as of local historic interest.

Her effects were sold, and the bed was bought by the then owner of Penfound Manor. With my previous knowledge, I was able to describe in more detail the 16th century bed. There at the head were small cupboards, which had held the Bible, personal weapons, and lastly, documents. The galleon had been either that of a Vice-Admiral or of a Senior Commander.

Penfound Manor was no longer open to the public when we left Poughill. If it is once more, a visit would be well rewarded. The north coast of Cornwall is notable for surfing. One day Rennie and I with Eva, and members of her family, were spending the day on the beach at Bude. I went surfing, and after a time, a current carried me a little further down the coast. Then riding on the crest of a roller, the surfboard hit a submerged rock. My bathing trunks were neatly severed, and all that remained was a long 'tail' stretching behind me. The beach was crowded, and I kept waving and shouting to Rennie to bring me a towel. She of course could not hear, and kept waving back. At long last I had to come out, and carrying the surfboard before me, with a long trail unwinding to the rear, I became a source of much banter and hilarious merriment not only to those of our own party, but of others, who could not conceal their interest in my modern substitute for a fig leaf. Rennie came to the rescue with an all enveloping towel and thus ended surf bathing for that day.

The idea of a visit to Paddy in the United States was ever present in our thoughts, and we decided to go as soon as we could manage it. There were no holiday charter companies then, as there are today, so we joined the North American Families Association, which was formed about that time, to facilitate family visits by members, both to and from the United States and Canada.

Paddy was living with her actor husband, John Wynne-Evans. We had seen him perform in England, when he played the lead in 'Waiting for Godot'. We were much impressed by his interpretation of such a difficult part.

Agatha Cristie's play the 'Mouse Trap' was to be produced in New York. One of the principal characters is described as 'A tall fair-haired Welshman speaking Welsh fluently'. This description fitted Paddy's husband, John, exactly. He applied for the part, but was turned down, as the New Yorkers' vision of a Welshman was of a short dark man. So the part was given to an Italian, whose broken American-English, spoken with an Italian accent, filled the bill to the satisfaction of the New York audiences.

This was a bitter blow to John's acting ambition.

Our first transatlantic holiday was to visit them in New York, where they had a flat in one of the old red brick buildings. They had made a charming home in unpromising surroundings. They had constructed small bay greenhouses outside of the long windows. This was a remarkable achievement in the heart of such a busy thriving city.

We explored so many parts of New York, that it is difficult to recall all that we saw, so long ago. Greenwich village was indeed noteworthy. I was impressed with the dock area and the huge wharves for the Atlantic liners, the Queen Mary, Queen Elizabeth, Normandie, and the present 'blue ribbon' holder, The United States. This era of the great passenger liners is a memorable one for many alive today.

"Oh to sit at the Captain's table."

My most vivid personal recollection is of our visit to the Morris-Jumal House. This Mansion was built in the colonial period in 1765. My forbears were closely associated with it. My son, Morris, is named after Col. Roger Morris, who married Mary Phelipse. Her sister, Susanne, married my ancestor Col. Beverley Robinson.

Unfortunately, it was near closing time, when we arrived with Paddy to go over the house.

An interesting piece of family history may have had some bearing on the political situation at the time.

Beverley Robinson, Roger Morris, and George Washington were brother officers under Gen. Braddock, during the successful war against the French in North America. Later, Mary Phelipse refused the hand of George Washington, and married Roger Morris. On arrival we were fortunate to be greeted by the Secretary of the 'Daughters of the Revolution'. When I mentioned to her that I was a descendant of Beverley Robinson, she became quite excited and said, "That was the cause of the trouble." She explained, "When George Washington proposed to Mary Phelipse and was refused, he never got over it." According to her, this disappointment finally decided him to break with England. However that may have been, Washington never forgot his friends of the past. My great-grandfather, Morris Robinson, was an officer in the King's Own Loyal Americans. Just before the surrender by Cornwallis, he was in a small outpost which was overrun by the 'rebels', and he was captured. When he declared he was an American, be was in great danger of being lynched. Washington heard about the situation however, and my great-grandfather was released. Later he returned to England and was posted to Gibraltar.

The Phelipse family was one of the wealthiest in New York. Frederick Phelipse was one of the founders of New Amsterdam, which later, by treaty, became New York. Mary Phelipse was indeed a wealthy woman, but on the conclusion of the war, all her property, then legally her husband's, was confiscated by the American government.

Most of the Loyalists either returned to England or moved to Canada.

Morris-Jumal Mansion had the rare distinction of being the only historic house in New York to be visited by Queen Elizabeth II and H.R.H. Prince Philip, at the time of the Bicentennial celebrations.

****

Soon after we returned home, we were distressed to hear that Paddy's marriage had become too stressful to continue, and they had decided to separate.

Paddy was teaching in New York. She found that her English qualification was not recognised in U.S.A. but was of accessory value. She studied for American diplomas and graduated well.

There was an advertisement for a teacher in California. Paddy applied for the post and was appointed. This meant a clean break with New York. She was faced with the difficulty of transporting her furniture, and other belongings, thousands of miles across the United States. Fortunately a friend of hers was delivering a truck to San Francisco. He and another mutual friend offered to take Paddy and all her belongings with them to San Francisco. She gladly accepted their help, and duly arrived to take up her new post.

She was not happy in her new surroundings. She learnt that she had been appointed as a 'WASP', White Anglo-Saxon-Protestant. In other words, rather anti-black, so she soon resigned and took another post in San Francisco associated with the children of immigrants. This was her real metier, and she has now retired after a most successful career.

Over the years, Rennie and I enjoyed three visits to San Francisco to see her. The first was through the American Families Association.

Among the presents we were taking on that occasion was a bottle of mead, pure Somerset brew.

On arrival at Gatwick airport, we were told that the time of the flight had been changed, and that the aircraft had left earlier. We had not been told, but everyone else had. Every effort was being made to find seats for us on another aircraft. We were fixed up at an hotel for the night, and we were assured that Paddy was being informed. We were told to be ready to leave as soon as seats on a flight could be arranged. Early next morning, we were informed that seats had been found for us on a flight from Heathrow.

A taxi was waiting for us, and almost before we had closed the door it was off. At Heathrow we were bundled out of the taxi, rushed through the check places, and our baggage seized, in spite of my determined effort to retain the holdall, which contained the mead. I uttered a warning that the bag contained a bottle of mead, which was fragile. "It will be all right" was the reply, and we found ourselves dumped, with our baggage, on a truck which tore towards a waiting aircraft.

It was a Pan-Am super plane. As we dismounted from the truck, I grabbed the holdall. When Rennie and I were ushered into the plane, it seemed as if all the passengers turned to gaze at us. It was then, that I became aware of a smell of mead, and the dampness of my trouser leg. The bottle had been broken and the intoxicating aroma of mead spread among the passengers. Never had we felt so self-conscious, and confused. The hostess seemed unconcerned, as though mead spillage was an everyday occurrence. She put us at our ease, and we tried to enjoy the flight.

We had let Paddy know the E.T.A. at San Francisco airport. The flight we were on terminated at Los Angeles, where we were to change for San Francisco and the last plane had left, which meant waiting at the airport until morning. Rennie by this time had a headache. Fumbling in the holdall, amid the mead residue, I managed to find the aspirin bottle. As I removed the cap, the bottle, which was slippery with mead, slithered from my grip, scattering aspirin tablets right and left. A young lad nobly gathered them all up, and handed them to Rennie. We thanked him profusely. Somehow the need for them had gone.

Paddy had received the first message from Gatwick, which she interpreted to mean that we were arriving at Los Angeles instead of San Francisco. So she drove over 200 miles to Los Angeles to find we were not there. Finally she left the airport and returned to her flat. By now I was confused as to the days and nights which had passed since leaving Heathrow. I rang Paddy to say we were arriving at San Francisco next morning. By this time Paddy and I were both so bewildered that she had doubts of my sanity. I was in no state to disabuse her! After a most uncomfortable night at Los Angeles airport, we caught the first flight for San Francisco. It was with profound thankfulness that we saw Paddy waiting for us, our anxiety was dissipated, as we, our relief unbounded, greeted each other. As for so called jetlag, it took us a long time to recover our equanimity.

At this distance in time I find it difficult to differentiate between all the holidays we had with Paddy.

One particular visit to Paddy's school on our first trip to San Francisco does stand out. She had made a large cut-out of an apple tree, which was affixed to the schoolroom wall. As the seasons changed she attached buds, then leaves and blooms, fertilised flower buds, and finally fruits, with the falling leaves of autumn.

She was devoted to her work, and her past pupils must have fond memories of her.

Our last visit was just before my 90th birthday, when Paddy gave such an enjoyable party, to which my nephew, Christopher, and his wife, Betty, came from the North West Territory of Canada!

Most unfortunately, this last visit was marred for Rennie, when the cornea of her right eye was abrased on replacing her plastic lens. This was the evening before leaving, and meant a hurried dash to her optician, who saw her at once and advised her to go to Moorfields Eye Hospital, as an emergency. It started to pour with rain when, at nearly 10p.m., Waring took us both in his car, and as speedily as he could, drove up the M10. The M10 was in a state of upheaval, with road widenings both at junctions with the M25 and the North Circular Road. In the pouring rain, which continued non-stop, and dense traffic, it was a nightmare drive, but Waring did manage to find Moorfields Eye Hospital. Greatly relieved after the strain of driving for Waring, plus the anxiety about our transatlantic flight next morning, Waring and I got out of the car. Then, as Rennie attempted to follow, she slipped and was wedged between the car and the kerb. Fortunately we saw the humour of the situation and laughed at the latest mishap as the clock struck 11p.m. We at last found the reception room, where we were expected. Rennie was seen at once by the emergency oculist, and to her and our relief, she was told that she could catch tomorrow's flight, but must do without her plastic lens until the abrasion was completely healed. Rennie had instructions to apply an ointment three times a day to the right eye. The rain had ceased and the drive back was free from anxiety.

We had time for only a few hours sleep before leaving for Gatwick. Morris had taken care to smooth the way for us however. As a result we received sympathetic help from everyone at the airport, and on the aircraft.

At San Francisco airport Paddy and her great friend, John Suscich, met us to our great relief. They had a wheelchair to help Rennie. Our anticipations were joyfully realised, when we saw Paddy's house. By then it was almost dark, all the lights were on, and it was so cheerful a welcome, and full of originality. The garden goes downhill in terraces, each level is called a 'deck'. It will be most attractive when she has accomplished all that she wants to do. There is a delightful conservatory, in which we spent a lot of our time.

On Tuesday, the 15th of July, Paddy took us to the Japanese garden in Golden Gate Park. It was a delightful experience, and in the Pavillion we had morning tea, Japanese style. Paddy went to fetch the car, whilst we sat on a comfortable seat, and watched the crowd pass by. Then we saw a sheriff on horseback ride up, he had a revolver clearly visible in its holster. Naturally we were all agog, but he was not there to arrest a violent criminal, but simply to plant a ticket on a parked car; very disappointing.

We were still suffering from jet lag, mixed with exhaustion following Rennie's unfortunate experience just before setting out. It was not until the fifth day that we felt really fit. On July 18th we had a lovely day. John Suscich invited us out to lunch, and we had a delicious meal of barbecued salmon, while Paddy had made a very tasty blackberry and apple pie. The journey to John's house was a delight, the route was over the Golden Gate Bridge and into Marin country. This is spectacular country of hills, and when clear, vistas over the bay and ocean.

After lunch John's friend, Bill, took us to see and explore a new American house; the price was only six hundred and twenty thousand dollars. It was a beautiful place, situated amidst marvellous scenery of woods and hills. We didn't make an offer! Bill then took us on a very pleasurable drive through breathtaking scenery, up the highest mountain overlooking the bay, where we watched the mist swirling over San Francisco, and so home to bed.

On the Sunday, Paddy took us to the wine country, which was most interesting. We bought some wine for Paddy's dinner party. This part of California is very rich in cultivation, it is much hotter than the coastal area, which is cooled by the Humbold current. There are numerous missions, and the Roman Catholic Church has achieved a great many conversions among the native population.

On Monday, we went with Paddy to the Science Museum. She left us there whilst she went to work and we had an enthralling time.

The Natural History Museum was beautifully set out, and in one part, to make it more realistic, they even provided the sounds of the birds and animals. Later we had a rather rummy lunch. We got it out of a self service contraption. We could not make out what was which, or what we got. I can only describe it as 'peculiar'. Then we went to the Planetarium, where in the dark we fell asleep.

Tuesday, and Paddy showed us a lot of San Francisco. It is a beautiful city, situated on many hills, with spectacular views. It is an offence to leave a car parked without turning the front wheels into the kerb, so as to avoid driverless runaways. We lunched on the waterfront in a pleasant restaurant.

Later we saw the other side of the city. The Chinese area might well be in a different country, there is such a variety of people and languages. It struck us too as being vibrant with life.

On Wednesday, while Paddy and I did some gardening, Rennie cooked us a superb lunch. Later, we all went to a garden centre and afterwards watched the Royal Wedding on television. Next day we did nothing very successfully, but later went to some friends of Paddy for dinner. Helen, a warm, vivacious woman, her husband and son, all welcomed us hospitably to their home. Later that evening, Paddy and I went to meet Christopher and Betty. The next day was, according to Rennie and Paddy, the day of days. It was to be an early celebration of my 90th birthday, as on the actual date, we would have returned home. About thirty guests arrived, who had known the house prior to Paddy's renovations, and were loud in their praises. Apart from her alterations and improvements, Paddy had blown up with helium gas about forty balloons, which floated and bobbed about the conservatory roof. It all looked very festive, then quite out of the blue, someone started singing "Happy birthday to you." I felt something of a fraud, anticipating my birthday which was still a month away.

Since a boy, I have collected stamps, and Paddy produced an enormous chocolate cake, decorated to look like a commemorative stamp with 'First Day of Issue' on it. An unusual and greatly appreciated birthday cake.

****

On one of our holidays with Paddy, her friend, John Suscich took the three of us for a tour along the Pacific coast. This area was famous, or rather, infamous, during the Prohibition period. John took us to a small restaurant perched on a cliff facing the ocean. This, he explained, was at one time a hide-out for Al Capone, who was a violent opponent of prohibition. He smuggled cargoes of intoxicants, to the bewilderment and fury of the excise officers.

He is always referred to as such a desperate character. However, there was another side to him which I learnt about from a patient of mine in Bexley, who had been a skipper of old sailing clippers, and was then a comrade in the anti-prohibition campaign. One day he and Al Capone were in a vessel running contraband liquor. Al Capone had taken advantage of the prevalent dense fog to attempt a landfall in secrecy, when the mist suddenly lifted, and his boat was exposed to the view of a customs launch some considerable distance away. The Customs Officer on the launch at once challenged Al Capone, ordering him to heave to. Al Capone, seeing the fog bank was still near, ignored the order, and at full speed made for the cover of the mist. The Customs Officer fired a shot, (whether as only a warning or not is unimportant), because Al Capone's vessel was hit, and began to sink, but not before it reached the comparative safety of the fog bank. My patient and Al Capone were struggling in the water, when, and here my memory cannot be absolutely certain, an inflatable dinghy was floating after the boat sank.

Al Capone found it, and having managed to get in, realised the custom's launch was methodically searching the area, but risked his hope of escaping by looking for his comrade, my patient, thereby jeopardising his own liberty. He continued seeking and finally found his companion in dire distress. He managed to get him into the dinghy, and thanks to the fog, evaded their pursuers and reached the shore. It may well have been his 'hide out', which was now our pleasant cafe.

Rightly or wrongly my patient would never bear a word against Al

Capone without being loud in his praises.

My patient had put a lot of his capital into the venture, and lost it all. Fortunately he was offered the task of sailing an old four masted sailing ship, manned by a skeleton crew, from San Francisco round Cape Horn to England. I saw a photograph of the ship, and heard his account of that grim voyage.

Financially it was a success, and enabled him to retire to Bexley.

I have always been a total abstainer, not originally as a matter of principle, but because I suffered from a a form of indigestion, which was painful, whenever I sampled wine as a boy. Since then I have been a teetotaller.

At Bexley I was asked to conduct a debate on 'Prohibition', and to speak on its behalf at the Freemantle Hall.

This was at the time when attempts were made to inforce it by law in the U.S.A. If ever there was a case of asking for trouble, this was it. Control of alcohol consumption can only be achieved by education.

The United States was such a vast country, with innumerable home brewing, apart from an enormously wealthy multinational industry of wines and spirits, that any hope of success through banning was doomed.

I would have preferred not to speak for prohibition, but for abstinence. However, I had no choice, so I wrote to the States for information. The amount of propaganda I received was huge. I do not think that I succeeded in reading all of it. The results of carefully recorded research on a scientific basis were incontestable.

The following facts demonstrate how alcohol is the great deceiver.

As a stimulant, this effect is transitory, and is due to stimulation of the nerve endings in the tongue.

Feeling of body warmth, due to flushing of the skin, with consequent loss of body heat. Sensation of acute perception and improved efficiency. On the contrary, careful measurement of reaction times shows delay of perception and reaction!

This last result is now well recognised in our law on drinking and driving. Yet it is present after even moderate consumption of alcohol.

As regards the debate, the result depended on the casting vote of the Chairman, who voted on behalf of his after dinner glass of port!

I do not think anyone nowadays would deny the futility of prohibition, but the attempt to enforce it left an extensive underground network as a likely source for Mafia like gangs to use for drug smuggling.

We will never know the full truth about this ghastly legacy.

Suddenly in the year 1968, the South Western Hospital Board realised that I was 74 years of age. The official limit for doing consultant locum work was 70, and so I was deprived of a source of income, and felt the loss of standing as a specialist. I was soon asked by a local general practitioner to act as his locum, and others followed suit. I enjoyed general practice once more, there is a personal relationship with a family, which is lacking in consultant work.

One patient I recall particularly, was an elderly widow. When I paid her a call, she ushered me into a world of dolls. I had never seen anything to compare with the immense variety of characters they represented. In what would have been otherwise a lonely existence, she lived in a world of make-believe. Yet she was not withdrawn, and it was always a visit I appreciated. Sadly, when I acted as locum for her doctor again, I heard that she had died. I have no idea what happened to her collection of such beautifully dressed and cared for progeny.

There was another patient I was asked to see who was a hermit. He lived in a small cottage, and when I entered the room where he was lying sick in bed, I had to thread my way through a multitude of old dry batteries. Originally, when he was fit, he had hoped to find a means of salving the constituents. Unfortunately he had a mild stroke, which severely incapacitated him, and the only part of his hoped for salvage was the ever increasing mass of exhausted dry batteries. He recovered from his bout of influenza, but in a year or two I saw his cottage for sale.

We had a wonderful fourteen years at Moorcroft, our very own home.

In 1972, Paddy hoped to make a change from her usual routine of coming to England, and spending her time visiting the family. We settled on a rather exciting holiday programme. We were to meet in Belgium, tour that country and elsewhere as the fancy took us, then back to England, before Paddy returned to San Francisco. Alas, it was not to be.

I discovered that vaccination against smallpox was imperative. So in good time I got vaccine, and vaccinated both Rennie and myself. All was going well, until one day my vaccinated area developed a secondary infection, and I had quite a high temperature. Our personal friend, the local G.P., called and put me on penicillin. My condition rapidly deteriorated, with the development of high fever, and I was covered with a virulent looking rash. Suddenly, I found myself in the fever hospital at Plymouth. By this time I was feeling terrible. When the consultant for infectious diseases saw me, and heard the history, he cancelled all antibiotics, for it seemed I was hypersensitive to penicillin.

From that moment I started to recover, and within a few days was able to return home, but our holiday plans had to be cancelled. My convalescence was prolonged and our eldest son, Waring, in particular was anxious that both his parents should be nearer to him.

He was also hoping to enlarge his home and had already approached the local authority for this purpose. He suggested that on account of my recent illness we should live closer to him. This had certainly been a great shock, and speaking for myself I could foresee future difficulties. In a year or two I should be eighty. I was still feeling weak, depressed and finding the gardening a strain. Waring offered to build us an annex to his house, as our permanent home.

Rennie was far from happy at the idea, it would be an agonising wrench for both of us to part with the lovely home we had spent so much time and energy in creating.

There was no member of our immediate family nearby. Of course Rennie's sister, Eva, and her daughter were only a few miles away. As regards our own children, Waring lived in Hertfordshire, Morris in Swindon, our eldest, Elizabeth, with her family, was in Guernsey, and Paddy in San Francisco. The value of our property had increased tenfold with all the improvements we had made during the years.

By selling, we could help Waring with his proposed extensions, also assist the others with smaller extensions which they had in mind.

Perhaps the deciding factor was that we were entering, in all probability, our last few years. Certainly I never expected to be writing my memoirs when 97 years old.

I made what I now feel was probably the wrong decision, and put Moorcroft up for sale, as in another few years its value would have trebled.

****

In December 1974 we moved from Cornwall to our new home, The Pightle Annexe, Hertingfordbury, Hertford.

The break from Cornwall was softened by having our family and especially the grandchildren, as daily companions.

How the history of our land is writ in the place-names of our country. Our new home was in Hertingfordbury, 'The fort on the ford protecting the town of Hertford'. Before the railways were reduced by Beeching, our small village had its own railway station, and, it was possible to travel through Hertford by train to anywhere in the United Kingdom. Now the branch line has gone, but its past still persists as a rural foot and pony trek. It is now a safe refuge for wildlife, birds, wayside flowers, and a haven for butterflies.

Our new home The Pightle, of which the Annex forms an addition, was built by an Anglo-Historian, who gave it this name, which in Anglo-Saxon means an irregular piece of enclosed land. In size it is about one third of an acre, and well wooded. It was and still is the home for many wild birds.

It was in late December when we first settled in, and we could look through the large sliding windows of our sitting room at the garden with its multitude of different trees.

At first, with the arrival of spring, the outlook was delightful, but as the trees became full leaf, our view became more and more circumscribed, until we felt as if we were living in Robin Hood's hide-out. The garden was really a small copse.

There was scope for both of us to help with the garden. The previous owner had had a bonfire site within full view of the bungalow. With the passage of years, it had grown to an unsightly heap. So with the approval of Waring and Alison, Rennie set to work with her usual energy, and in short time levelled it, and made a fresh site the other side of the copse. As I was so near my eighties, I had not considered taking on locum work, and assumed that my medical career was over. Fate had other ideas, however, and thereby hangs this tale.

My son, Waring, was in general practice in Hertford, and as the practice was largely rural, visits could be at a distance. At that time he was a lone practitioner, but a number of the doctors in Hertford took turns for emergencies.

One day, a Dr. Robertson was 'on call' when a woman, some miles away, collapsed with heart failure in her cottage.

Unfortunately, Dr. Robertson had been called to an emergency elsewhere. Waring was the next on the rota, but he was attending another case and could not leave at once. I decided to go myself, and see what the old man could do to tide over the period until the patient could be got to hospital. I still had my emergency kit, and I hurried off to see if I could help this unfortunate woman. Luckily when I found the cottage, which was one of a terrace, the front door was ajar and I went in.

It was obvious the patient was desperately ill, and I asked a neighbour to send for the ambulance whilst I did what I could to help her. Just as I was preparing an injection, Dr. Robertson arrived. He was equipped with all the modern emergency kit, and took over the treatment.

Naturally I withdrew, and waited in the background.

As Dr. Robertson administered an injection, the patient was showing some improvement when the ambulance arrived, and she left in it for hospital.

Dr. Robertson thanked me for my effort and left. Although I had not given an injection to the patient, I had already sterilised my syringe and was about to do so, when Dr. Robertson arrived, fully prepared for immediate action and of course with the modern throw away technique.

Every one had gone and I was alone in the cottage, with a little clearing up to do, and my bag to pack, before I left. When I went to open the front door, I found it was locked, and there was no key. I decided to try the back door. This had also been locked, and I could find no key to that one either.

When, one is inadvertently locked inside a cottage, it is surprising how difficult it can be to attract attention to one's marooned state.

The windows were tiny and to attempt to escape that way would be hazardous.

I examined the locks on the front and rear doors. The front one could be removed, if the necessary tools were to hand. I had just the things in the car, but that of course was far out of reach. I searched the kitchen and elsewhere. The only tools I could find were a corkscrew and a tin opener. From my bag I took a pair of Spencer-Wells artery forceps, and thus equipped started to attempt to unscrew the locks. The back door lock wouldn't budge, but the front door was more tractable. There was some give in one screw and I managed to unscrew it, then I was able to move the whole lock slightly and gradually free the other screws, and finally with relief the door was open. I had escaped but how to shut the door was the question now. Finally I jammed it with a thick wad of paper, and sped off home in the car.

Happily, the patient recovered sufficiently to return to her home. I had left the screws to the front lock in a prominent spot, carefully replacing the corkscrew and tin opener.

At the Pightle, I considered pruning the trees, so that in summer we could do more than get just a glimmering of the sky. At the same time, I ordered some fruit trees to add to the small orchard in the front garden. Rennie made a charming rockery outside our sitting room window, which was on a mound. Unfortunately a May tree grew on the mound and its branches spread so close to the wall of the annex that it had to be dug out. Afterwards its roots sent up shoots which were hard to eradicate.

During the Second World War, a German plane had jettisoned its load of bombs on the garden. Nature, the sculptor of time, had turned the craters and mounds into attractive diminutive valleys and hillocks. Wild flowers grew in profusion. Every spring, the first harbingers were the golden celandines peeping through their sward of deep green leaves. Then soon to follow there would be a haze of blue reminiscent of our lost Dartmoor beauty spot, followed later by primroses which girdled the shrubs and trees. In quiet seclusion, the umbellaria raised their bell-shaped flowers. Later the garden was alight with masses of daffodils.

Besides ourselves in the annex, there were other newcomers. When on holiday in Yorkshire, Waring and Alison bought a puppy. She was a Border collie, and became a loved family pet. The family decided to call her Floss, so I promptly announced "She will be 'Candy' to me." A quip which did not seem to amuse the others.

Alison added to the family pets two ducks and a drake. What different characters our new pets had! Of course the puppy, Floss, was at first rather shy and withdrawn, and she would seek the seclusion of her lair under the window seat in the kitchen. Hunger induced her to take an interest first in food, then in those who offered it. Soon, after one or two tentative approaches, her tail rose, and began to wag. From then on, relieved of fear, her trust and devotion grew rapidly. Our grandchildren adored her, and the girls had an amusing time rounding up the ducks, when Floss hugely enjoyed herself barking fussily, and causing confusion to the raucous indignation of his lordship the drake. I felt this to be a pity, as the inbred sense of a Border collie for rounding up sheep might be lost. Far from it, for on one occasion Rennie was alone in the house, when she suddenly spotted the ducks loose in the front garden, with an open way into the public road. The gate from the kitchen yard had not been shut. Rennie called Floss, and said quietly "Floss go fetch them." Floss with no fuss bypassed the errant ducks, then quietly drove them to and through the kitchen yard gate. True she did not close it, but left that duty for Rennie. Floss earned her praise, for what a tragedy it would have been for the girls to find their pets lost, when they returned from school.

When I first retired, Rennie and I decided to buy a motor caravan, if we could afford one. We heard of one called The Debonair, supplied by a firm at Folkestone, and decided to go to view one. Our arrival happened at a fortunate time for us. There was the very model which had been on show at Olympia. Since then, the firm had toured Europe with it for demonstration purposes. The vehicle had been in some of the roughest mountain terrain, and was on offer at a bargain price. We did not hesitate, but bought it at once. The layout was remarkable. Extra space in front was obtained by the gear change being on the steering column. The front seat was a bench and its back could fold down to form a double bed. The rear seats did likewise, so there was sleeping accommodation for four. The centre of the van housed the cooking stove, fridge and cupboards. All this in a Bedford light C.A.V. van.

We had this vehicle for over twenty years, and toured the United Kingdom, Ireland, and the Continent. We would have it today, but for a desperate accident on the M4 motorway.

We were travelling westwards, approaching the turn for Slough, when from the rear came a terrific roar, and the car was flooded with a blazing glare. With a crash we appeared to be airborn, then tipped on end, our seat-belts saving us from being catapulted out as the car, now nearly vertical, travelled forwards on its front wheels. With a hesitant balance, it teetered slowly backwards, and then ponderously lurched down on to four wheels. At first I thought a plane had crashed, but all was now comparatively quiet.

It was dusk and to add to our perplexity, it was the rush hour. Traffic was zooming home, both along the M4 and to Slough. At first, Rennie and I were in a state of shock. As soon as I had recovered enough, I opened my door and got out, finding myself engulfed in the noise and lights of homing vehicles. Flattened against the side of our van, I could see no vehicle immediately behind. When I managed to reach the rear, I found a large headlight embedded within our rear door, and the whole back of the caravan was pushed inwards.

The Slough turning was about twenty yards behind. I could see a number of lorries parked in the distance down towards Slough. The culprit could have been there. I attempted to cross the road, but it was obvious that to do so was impossible with the continuous stream of traffic.

Returning to the wagon, I suggested to Rennie that we would see if the car could still travel. To our surprise the engine started and the vehicle was mobile and responding to steering. We had been on our way to Morris at Abingdon, so we decided to continue cautiously, and have the damage assessed at the nearest garage. We also notified the police, who, as soon as they heard that no one was injured, were not interested.

I had a fully comprehensive insurance when I bought the van, but when its value had dropped, due to the passage of fifteen years, I changed to a third party one. Hence the insurance company was uninterested, unless I could identify either the culprit or his vehicle. The old question "Did you take his number?" was repeatedly asked.

Apart from what had happened to the rear door, the full extent of the damage was not realised until the chassis revealed resultant fatal flaws. These came to light when our vehicle was due for its next M.O.T. test. I was asked to call at the garage as soon as possible. Everybody there well knew what a treasured possession our motor caravan was, and a very grim faced mechanic, usually so pleased to see me, silently beckoned me to come with him. He showed me that the main chassis had on the offside a huge gap where the girder had fractured, it was a gap of several inches, through which one's hand could easily pass. Other parts of the chassis were cracking, and the damage was too severe for repair.

The old M.O.T. certificate had not expired, so driving cautiously, I went to a dealer with a view to buying another motor caravan and expecting to be allowed something in part exchange. I was certainly taken aback when the salesman refused the part exchange, but offered me a £100 off the price of another, if I took our van, of so many treasured memories, out of his sight. This convinced me that our motor caravan was definitely a wreck. I accepted his offer and bought another, which though faster, had not the same comforts.

****

Our Debonair had been a home, during specialist locums in Wales and Ulster. The last locum in Belfast had ended just before the present 'troubles' started.

The loveliest holiday Rennie and I had enjoyed in it was in Wales, and I cannot do better than quote from the notes Rennie made at the time. The year would probably have been 1968.

"Sept. 9th. First day of holiday has arrived. We intended starting early, but I had a bad night, so we did not leave until 10a.m. First to Hertford, to the office of the Mercury local paper, to arrange a time for a photograph of our grandson, Magnus, with his 15ft sunflower. We were surprised at the pleasure and eagerness shown to hear our story about the Children's Society and the scheme for people to sponsor the growth of the Sunflower at twopence an inch.

Back to the Pightle and Alison's welcome "What have you forgotten this time?"

By midday we were away, the weather was bright and so were our spirits. We are both gypsies at heart, and the thought of a wandering holiday always delights us. We made very good time to Shrewsbury and stopped at Nestcliff, a lovely camp where we stayed two years ago when Paddy was at a summer college near Shrewsbury.

Sept. 10th. A lovely morning and we are happily on our way to Wales. It was a marvellous run and soon we were in the hills. What beautiful country! We got to Porthmadoc about 4p.m. and then on to Morfa Bychan two miles further on. In vain we looked for the Morfa Bychan we knew in 1947. Now, it is one vast caravan and chalet park.

We did not have much trouble in finding a camp, had our tea and decided to go for a walk to find part of Morfa we could recognise. Alas nothing, until we got to the beach, that vast sandy stretch with a background of hills had not changed, and we returned to our camp and bed.

Next morning, the 11th, a very damp awakening, rain, rain and yet more rain. We did go for a walk, but not to the hills. On the other side were lovely winding walks and some quite rare shrubs and trees. We found a grotto which Magnus, our grandson, would have loved. We had lunch in the car, then a snooze. Later we found the telly a great boon and, our Calor gas fire kept us beautifully warm. We saw some blue sky and the rain had gone, so we decided to go for a stroll to see if we could find a chalet, or caravan suitable for Waring and family. Most of the camps here let plots for people who own their own caravans or chalets. We became very interested in a caravan for sale, £3,300.00, sleeping six and everything provided, £300 extra to have electricity, main water and drainage. Easy to get the money back by letting, but we gave up the idea as we thought it unwise to tie ourselves up at our time of life. Still it would have been lovely to have a place of our own so near the sea and mountains. During the afternoon we went to Porthmadoc to shop, and found it was closing day. However, Geoffrey managed to buy a lemon squeezer. (I forgot to mention that on the A1 we stopped to buy oranges, 100 for £1, we couldn't resist such a juicy offer. Hence the lemon squeezer).

We went to the bank and cashed a cheque. Geoffrey having taken the squeezer from me went and left it at the bank. We also asked about the trains on the Festinog railway.

Sept. 12th we decided to go to Portmeirion, it is only about three miles from Porthmadoc. To get in, we had to pay 65p each reduced rate for O.A.Ps. It certainly is a remarkable place and whoever was the architect must have been a great lover of Italy. It is beautifully situated on a small peninsular, and on that day the sun shone, so we enjoyed the colourful houses and gardens with statuary. The best part was looking over a small inlet of Tremadoc bay, with a view of the hills on the other side.

Today is Festinog Railway day, I forgot to say that we rescued the lemon squeezer from the bank. We arrived at the station to catch the 11 o'clock train and, as it was a Saturday, the train did not leave 12 noon. To kill time we went to the Maritime museum. Geoffrey enjoyed it, while I trailed after him and tried to feel some interest in rusty pieces of boat equipment and Victorian photos. The weather was dull but dry, so we looked forward to our trip on the small gauge railway. We found comfortable seats and the sound of the engine brought back childhood memories of steam trains. We chugged through the hills higher and higher, stopping at small halts, and ascending all the time. The views were very beautiful, and when we got to our destination we were allowed ten minutes to look around us. When we got back into the train, our seats had been taken, and we had a bit of a scramble to find others. Altogether it was a most interesting experience.

Sunday, the 15th, a sunny day and we decided to walk to Borth-a-Gest. I packed a lunch, and we walked across the firm sand for about a mile. When we turned the corner, there was the Borth-a-Gest we remembered, a beautiful bay, slate rocks, and sand hills. The season being over, there were very few people about. Some were boating or water-skiing. We sat on the sand with slate rocks for a backrest and enjoyed our lunch. Afterwards we went for a further walk, and eventually returned, walking again over the sands back to our camp. We decided to go for a run to find our way to Borth-a-Gest by road. The car refused to start, we had run the battery down using the T.V. Geoffrey turned and turned the starting handle, but not a spark of life. We decided to go to the garage to see if we could borrow a battery. Nothing doing, being Sunday, only one man was on duty and no spare battery. The garage attendant was chatting with a hefty local young man, and I decided to ask him for help.

"You look a likely strong man, could you give us a hand winding the car?"

He looked a bit surprised, but came back to the car. With a few good pulls the engine sprang to life and all was well. Our useful friend refused any refreshment.

Then we went for a run to put some life into the battery then back to camp and bed.

Monday the 15th. This morning the rain was pelting down, so we decided to go to Blaenau Festiniog to see the Llechwedd Slate caverns. By the time we got there the rain had more or less ceased. Those mountains of slate are amazing, we booked for the railway to the caverns. This is the largest slate quarry in the world. It was an unusually exciting trip, and we were impressed with the huge caverns. Our engine driver guide gave us a summary of the history and tools used. He had a soft Welsh voice and it was rather difficult to catch all he said, perhaps it was we who were 'hard of hearing'. After the railway, we went by cable-car to see the caverns. We had been impressed by the railway, but the caverns were even more wonderful and cathedral-like in height and construction. The depth, where we were, was about 800 ft., and there were more galleries underneath. We had to wear steel helmets, as some of the passages were rather low. To add to our pleasure, a harp was playing delightful music.

Then we came to a simply enormous cavern, hundreds of feet across and in height, it was lit up in different places showing the colours of the rock. There was a protective rail to stop us from falling into a large underground lake, the reflection of the rocks and lights made it a most beautiful sight, and this time our music was a full orchestra. I wish I knew the name of piece they were playing, it was lovely. To think that those caverns had been made by Victorian man, with small tools and dynamite. They put off the electric light, to give us an idea what it would be like working there. Then we saw, halfway up the rock-face, perched on a ledge, a Welshman, his only light a candle flame, singing in a wonderful tenor voice, which echoed and re-echoed around the cavern. The scene was reflected in the mirror of the lake. We have enjoyed our day and are very impressed with the way in which it was presented.

Tuesday 16th. We thought that yesterday was wet, but today the rain just lashed, down and we felt 'enough is enough' and regretfully agreed to return home. However we decided to see more sights and as Harlech, where the craft village called Maes Artrowas was on our way back, we had a look at it. Once more we were very impressed with the village and all the various things shown. We bought some woollens and tried to get a slate house sign for Waring. The man who made them was not there, so we left our address and telephone number, and we were assured he would get in touch with us.

It has turned out a lovely evening and we have stopped for the night in the heart of the mountains, Dolgelly Pass.

It is quite beautiful and we look forward to waking up tomorrow morning to such a view."

Rennie's notes of this memorable holiday ended here. In due course, we heard from the craftsman engraver and he made an admirable slate house sign 'THE PIGHTLE', which now hangs proudly on Waring's front door.

Wales is a fascinating country and full of surprises. When our first born was a baby, we were driving over the mountains to Festiniog, when we found the road completely filled with a crowd of folk singing their hearts out as they sped a bride and bridegroom away on their honeymoon. Their arms were linked and they almost frisked as they walked with unrestrained happiness filling us with a sense of exhilaration.

The mountains and valleys of Wales, with the lakes and streams, are the source of this mystic Celtic harmony. It is no wonder that the Welsh have an inborn sense of poetical concord, which we English so much admire.

****

At the Pightle I missed my greenhouse, so at first I had a small lean-to attached to the garden shed. This did well for tomatoes, but I missed having the space to grow grapes and peaches. At the far end of the garden I put up two greenhouses, one professional, and one added mainly from the lean-to. I was then able to grow seedlings for planting out. These had to be protected not only from slugs and other pests, but after a similar experience to one I had in Cornwall, from, of all birds, the humble wren.

One day in Cornwall when I opened the door into the greenhouse, there was a panic stricken wren fluttering about and causing untold damage among my seedlings. I opened the door wide and the window as well, but the intruder refused to leave and eventually huddled down in a corner among some flowerpots. I left it alone for some time, but when I returned, there it still was, again stricken with fear, as I approached. Eventually, when it huddled down, I managed to catch it. Taking it out into the garden, I opened my hand expecting it to fly away at once, but it appeared paralysed with fright. I gently stroked its head and then it perked up, and with a "chirrup" it flew off. To my surprise this performance was repeated again in a few days time. I did not have as much difficulty in catching the bird, and it flew away quicker on this occasion with its "chirrup." In about a week, back it came a third time, this occasion making no frantic attempt to escape, but waiting to be picked up, and away it flew, not forgetting its farewell "chirrup."

Now here at the Pightle I was faced with a similar incident. What is extraordinary is that history repeated itself. One morning in the larger greenhouse, I was faced with the frenzied panic of a wren, as it flew and scurried hither and thither. Again I opened the door and ventilator, tried to coax it out to freedom, but in vain. I left the glasshouse, and did some gardening. When I returned, the wren had not left, so I tried to catch it, and at last succeeded as it cowered in a corner. Once outside I opened my hand as I had previously done in Cornwall, and as then, the wren did not appear to realise it was free, but remained lying on the palm of my hand. I stroked its head and it apparently came to its senses and flew off with a "chirrup."

On the 'third' occasion, when it trespassed within the greenhouse, there was no effort to escape, it waited to be picked up and freed once more, with its cheery good-bye "chirrup."

I do not know the favourite diet of a wren, but I think that it is probably small insects, as I have never been able to entice one to feed from my hand. Wrens appear to be very timid, which makes my two experiences of their behaviour, one in the South-West in Cornwall, and the other in the home counties in Hertfordshire, so interesting.

Robins, who are soon willing to feed from one's hand, have a varied diet, as do sparrows, blackbirds and starlings. Our bird table proved a haven for tits. The grey squirrels were a menace and a constant campaign had to be kept up to protect the nesting birds from them. Floss made every effort to catch them. She succeeded only once, yet she never gave up trying.

Rennie and I were at the Pightle for eighteen years. A lot happened during the first twelve months. Alison had her first baby, Magnus, and so soon it seemed he was a toddler. He thought a lot of his grandmother, who, if his mother was busy, sang lullabies to send him to sleep, thus he called his granny 'Lallie', and Lallie she became to Magnus's two young sisters, Chloe and Esme, to all at the Pightle, as well as to neighbours.

In what seemed only a few years, Magnus was at preparatory school age. I vividly recall his first appearance in school uniform. There was the school cap, and such a wee Magnus underneath.

His development appeared so rapid to us, his grandparents. He was surprisingly skilled in origami. He made, as if by magic, numbers of amazing folded paper birds and animals. The door and walls of his small bedroom were covered with examples of midget paper puppets of fauna past and present. One day a notice was pinned to his door, which, to the amusement of the whole family, read, "Do not disturb, genius at work." Magnus was so under the spell of his progeny of mystical paper puppets that he was impelled to compose the following:-

"In my Granny's garden there are dinosaurs and things, Rats and bats and lizards which all have great big wings. In my Granny's garden the giraffe peeps over the wall. He chews the bark off trees because he's very tall!"

His young sisters, Chloe and Esme, first shared a double-bunk bed but they soon demanded separate beds.

Chloe, encouraged by her mother, developed her musical talent. She had an excellent music teacher, under whose care she did well She looked forward to his lessons. Then one day he did not come.

He had died from a heart attack. Chloe was so distressed, this was her first experience of the finality of death. In her anguish at the age of twelve, she wrote this sad lament:

'My Music Teacher'

Why did it have to happen ?
I mean why did he have to die.
He had a gift at the piano,
And was sharing it with me.

My piano teacher was old with white hair,
He was so kind and generous,
And I liked him so much.
Why did it have to happen?

If someone was to talk about it,
I'd feel upset, but not cry,
A brave face would come across me,
And I would bottle it up inside.

When I am in bed tonight,
I shall think of him until I sleep,
Why did he have to do it to me,
I mean, why did he have to die?

(Chloe Robinson.)

Christopher, Elizabeth's third child, is happily married and his wife, Julie, is his ardent partner in charitable works. They cater especially for deprived children by giving them holidays on the Norfolk Broads in motor boats, which Christopher and Julie have purchased for that purpose. Their effort has been so successful that they have been awarded a prize of £1,000 to extend and continue their scheme.

Elizabeth's youngest, Denise, and her husband Steven, are at present sharing Elizabeth's and Kenneth's home. They have a baby, John, and hope to find a house of their own soon.

Our grandchildren therefore are either adults, or soon will be, some are at universities, the youngest are still at school.

Our second child, Patricia, has already figured in this series of memoirs and she, in the course of her life, has been an example of triumph over adversity. She has made many friends in San Francisco, but I am sure that at heart she thinks longingly of the land of her birth.

How different children are even in the same family. Esme also has an ear for music, but she, in addition, has an affinity with animals and birds. They quickly sense this rapport, and she has many pets in the wild.

Where did these gifts come from? Alison has a deep love of music both instrumental and vocal. Waring always had a desire to excel in woodwork. During his spare time he has developed a craftsmanship which has won for him gold medals, crystal bowls and other prizes. Now that he is of retiring age he intends to spend his time perfecting his flair for developing the hidden beauty of the delicate intrinsic grain of different woods.

Meanwhile the greenhouses were producing grapes and peaches, and in a few years would have done well, but in the late eighties, one the worst hurricanes ever known in the British Isles did untold damage throughout the country. Thousands of trees were uprooted, roads were blocked, and numerous areas were flooded. At the Pightle, some of the trees in the copse were blown down, and my greenhouses severely damaged. I tried to repair them but I was already in my nineties and could not persevere, as I would have once been able to do.

By this time the need arose for extra room for our grandchildren. It was then we realised that we had far exceeded our allotted span of threescore years and ten!

So we eventually decided to leave the Pightle and retire to a home for the elderly.

So here we are today in the Cotswolds at the town of Witney, in a home for the elderly. We have kept some of the smaller articles of our old furniture.

Everyone here is most kind, but we miss the independence of our own home, and the company of our eldest, Waring, and our daughter-in-law, Alison, and their children, Magnus, Chloe, and Esme. They visit whenever they can. We have frequent visits from, and excursions with, our younger son, Morris, and Barbara, his wife, also Sarah, their daughter, and Simon, both now adults and doing well in the realm of higher education. When Simon was six years of age, he and a little girl, Fiona, were great chums and this friendship lasted for three years, when different schools parted them. I hoped in some way to commemorate this so simple and trusting friendship. An idea suggested itself to me. Both their homes were and still are in Abingdon, which is on the Thames. So I decided to build a model of a Thames barge, call it 'Fiona', port of origin Abingdon. I obtained a scale plan of a Thames barge and so was able to build a two foot model, plank on plank. Rennie made a set of sails, and now about twelve years later it is a memento of their past friendship. Fiona is now married but still lives in the neighbourhood.

Our daughter Elizabeth, is enjoying life with her husband, Kenneth, in Guernsey. Of their children, Suzanne, the eldest, is pressing on with further studies, and we her grandparents, will soon be very much out of date!

William, their second child, is now well placed in the senior nursing ranks of the Health Service. He and his wife, Sally, have two children, Charlotte, and a boy, Timothy.

My wife, Rennie, is now well into her 94th year, and her love through our 68 years of marriage has been the guiding influence for each member of our family, and will continue so for generations yet to come.

Now at 97 years of age, I end my memoirs conscious of the many errors I have made in the past, but thankful for all the blessings life has bestowed on my wife and myself.

AUTOBIOGRAPHY LOIS M I ROBINSON nee PAYNE.

Now that I have reached the age of 92. I must give way to the family's suggestion that I write a few of my reminiscences before my memory has really forsaken me. Where to begin? That is the problem.

My first memory of home and family was trying to sit on my Mother's knees and being firmly removed by Father, the reason being that my Mother was expecting another baby, and that meant that I would no longer be the youngest in the family. I remember so well when he was born, Father calling out "Come to see your brother." My two sisters, Violet and Eve, came rushing past me, and there was my Mother looking so lovingly at us and bending down to show us our brother. That was a very happy moment and will always remain in my memory, though so much else has faded.

We lived at the top of a very large house in Dublin. This was the top flat of the Irish Church Mission School. The Mission was started during the potato famine and Father was the Headmaster. The day started with breakfast being given to about one hundred children. That consisted of a mug of cocoa and hunks of bread and sometimes fruit. Poverty was extreme in the beginning of the 20th century. The Mission Homes were started by the Smiley family and were called the Smiley Homes. I believe that the Barnado Homes were run on the same principles. The school and Home were run by the Irish Church Mission which was of course Protestant. We had a very happy home life. except that Mother was ill on and off. She had never really recovered from typhoid fever a year before her marriage, and had not regained her strength before having babies. She caught the infection while visiting ill children belonging to the school. Dublin was not a very healthy place to live in at that time. We lived near to Phoenix Park, a lovely park with miles of woodland, hills and valleys. If my parents ever had the time to spare, we all watched polo being played by the Army, which then of course was the British Army, and the Gentlemen of Ireland. I particularly remember their lovely red coats and wishing Father was a soldier so that he could wear one.

We always had wonderful holidays. Dublin has lovely seaside places so near. Father used to rent a cottage and we lived almost in the sea. Mother would improve in health and that made us all happy. I remember very vividly one holiday at a small town called Skerries. As a great treat we were all, and by all I mean Father, Mother, my Uncle Finn (a nickname) and us four children. Seven in all started off on a sunny afternoon feeling very happy and full of life, the ages of us children were seven, five, three and a half, and baby a few months old. This was a trip in a boat, it was a very warm day. I got sleepy and was put in the bottom of the boat.

I was awakened by a big mouthful of salt water. I started to cry, and saw Father using his oar to push us away from rocks. Uncle Finn was swimming alongside and pulling the boat along. It was a very slow process as by now it was raining in torrents. In the distance we saw a small island which was very rocky and difficult to get to. However with much effort we did land and saw a broken down cottage with only a small piece of roof, under which we all crouched. Mother was very anxious about the baby, so Father and Uncle Finn collected bits of twigs and sticks and succeeded in making a fire. Father smoked a pipe so we had matches. The warmth comforted us a little.

Presently we heard voices calling to us. Some men from the village had seen us leave, and when the storm came, they felt that we would be in difficulties. They launched their boat to look for us. It was so good of them, and our relief and joy were great. As far as I can remember we were none the worse for our alarming experience.

My Grandfather, who was an Evangelist and a great Christian, was taking a mission service in Wales practically opposite Skerries. It was a prayer meeting, quite suddenly he said, "Friends, I have a feeling my family in Ireland is in great trouble. Let us pray for them." God answered his prayer and we were saved.

Ever since I have always had a fear of small open boats. Soon after we had returned home Mother's cough grew much worse and the doctor said we must move out of the city. Father found a house some way out of Dublin, and we soon moved there. What I remember most about it was the small garden, and the fun we had playing in it. There had been no garden at the school, but we played in the big empty school rooms. Another school had to be found for us three girls, our ages were Violet 8, Eve 5, and I was 4. I had always felt nervous about going to a proper school and was always getting into trouble for talking and making a noise. However we soon settled down and began to like our new life.

Mother did not improve in health. We had a daily woman in to help, she was very kind, but puzzled us by keeping on asking Mother the time. Her name was Mrs Looby. I asked Mother why does Mrs Looby keep asking the time when there is a clock in the kitchen? Mother replied that Mrs Looby could not tell the time. This so shocked us that we would chant "Mrs Looby is a great big booby, because she cannot tell the time."

Mrs Looby almost left, but Mother persuaded her to stay. Mother did not improve, in fact she became much worse and her coughing became awful, and then she had to stay in bed all the time. My Grandmother and Aunty Lois took it in turns in coming from Manchester and then to Dublin to look after us. It was a very distressing time for all of us, especially Father. Grandmother was a very emotional Welsh woman, and made us realise the possibility of Mother's early death. She taught us to sing a very poignant verse:-

"When I was a little child, how well I recollect
How I would grieve my Mother
With folly and neglect
But now that she has gone to Heaven
I miss her tender care
Oh Saviour, "Tell my Mother I'll be there!"

Mother was upstairs and I can still hear say, "Wait until I have gone." She had a great sense of humour.

Gradually Mother got much worse and we were told that she was leaving us to go to Heaven. I remember that one evening we all went in to say goodbye to her. She was so thin and looked so fragile. She had lovely brown eyes and very flushed cheeks. We were not allowed to kiss her, but she held our hands and looked so lovingly at us. That was the last time we saw Mother alive and it was the end of our home life. I was eight at the time.

What to do with four young children was a problem that had to be faced. It was decided that Lello (my brother Llewellyn) should go at once to Manchester to our paternal Grandparents and Aunty Lois. We three girls were to follow later. We spent about two weeks at the Y.W.C.A., where everyone was very kind to us. Then until we could go to Manchester we would stay at one of the Smiley homes (called The Bird's Nest). This filled us with dismay, and so began the worst three months of our lives. They were kind to us, but the difference from our home life was too much for me. I developed a bad cough which seemed impossible to cure, and I remember crying myself to sleep every night. Eve became very quiet and did not make friends with anyone. Violet spent her time telling people how different this life was from being at home.

After three months of misery Father came for us and took us all to Manchester. We had a loving welcome from our Grandparents, and our three Uncles. Uncle Finn was in his twenties, David was about sixteen and Ben was fourteen. They were tolerant and on the whole they were kind. Finn was particularly so, and I remember he made me a doll's cot. We soon settled down, then school for us had to be found, and as there was very little money, it had to be State education.

My first impression of School in Manchester was terrifying as I could not understand a word the children said, and they laughed when I spoke to them; they spoke broad Lancashire and I had an Irish brogue. My teacher was a lovely woman with such a kind face, she liked my Irish accent. Mother had taught us to read at a very early age. She too had been a teacher. Miss Lea, our teacher, would get me to read aloud, in the hope I think that the class would speak Lancashire with an Irish brogue!

Our life with our Grandparents was rather strict, and we were brought up on the saying 'Children should be seen and not heard'. The day started with family prayers immediately after breakfast. Grandfather read from the Bible, then we all knelt down and he would ask anyone he chose to say a word of prayer. That was terrible for us, Eve was struck dumb when she was chosen. All she could finally utter was, "Keep Father on the straight and narrow path." When my turn came and I was asked for a word of prayer, I crept very quietly out of the dining room on my knees!

Grandfather wrote religious books when he was not taking missions. He went to America three times and he was well liked. One of the American universities made him a Doctor of Divinity

(D.D.). In fact Grandfather was to America what Billy Graham was to England later on in the 20th century.

I remember on one occasion I had left my homework exercise book open on the table. Grandfather saw an open space on the page, whereupon he wrote one of his thoughts for fear of forgetting it. He would probably have included it in one of his books.

Next day at school a very stern voice from my teacher called "Rennie Payne come out!" I got up wondering whatever I had done this time. "What have you written in your homework?" Looking down I saw Grandfather's handwriting and realised that he had written a 'thought'. I replied to my teacher, "That is one of my Grandfather's thoughts." I was not reprimanded but told to keep my homework out of Grandfather's way. I did not do well at that school. My sisters Violet and Eva settled down and worked much better. I talked too much and in consequence spent much of my time at school outside the classroom door.

The highlight in our lives at that time was when Father came to England to spend his holiday, and I remember feeling jealous when I thought that he spent too much of his time with our uncles.

I have not said much about Aunty Lois, we could not have remained with our Grandparents if she had not been there. She was the backbone of the family, for the house was a big rambling one, which she ran very efficiently. Certainly we three girls thought so.

Grandmother was a real country woman, she was steeped in country lore. She had a remarkable knowledge of herbs, their medicinal qualities and uses. She did most of the cooking and made wonderful bread. I can still see the bread coming out of the oven in the wall. The smell was lovely and so appetising. I recall on one of our holidays in Anglesey we were having a picnic and found that our bottle of water was broken. There was no habitation where we were, and my Grandmother, who had a water diviner's instinct, without hazel rods, said "I will try to find some." It was a very rocky island with a lighthouse some way out to sea. Grandmother peered and examined the rocks in different places and chose one. She asked us to start digging in the sand close to the rock. We all set to and at last the sand began to get damp, then we all used our children's spades with energy and soon the hole began to fill with water. Grandmother told us to leave the hole alone for a short time. When we came back there was a clear pool of fresh water. I believe that the lighthouse people use the well that Grandmother found instead of walking four miles to a village to get their water. I remember they used donkeys for this purpose. The water was carried in two panniers, one on each side of the donkey.

Aunty Lois made all our clothes. She was a wonderful dressmaker. Life went on quietly until Grandfather and Uncle Finn started arguments about biblical matters, and I can still remember the heated discussions about evolution. They were both big men and they had a depressing effect at times.

However, a much more depressing cloud gradually came into our lives. Father wrote to tell us that he had become engaged to a woman called Lily Marshall, and that he was looking for a house to be our home. We were happy at the idea of a new home but not the idea of a stepmother.

Eventually he found an old Irish house just outside Dublin.

It had an enormous garden with a big coach house at the end of it. The garden was a delight to us, especially to Lello and me. We had great fun in it and we could climb on top of the coach house. From there we watched the recruits for the 'Republican' army drilling. We used to shout down to them "Call yourselves soldiers! You should see the British army drilling!" They took very little notice of us, but our behaviour did have one serious result. When the rebellion started Father was picked up by some Republican soldiers and taken to their headquarters in Clontarf, where he was questioned for hours. A neighbour of ours heard of his arrest. She knew the Officer in charge and assured him that Mr. Payne was quite innocent and that he must be freed to return to his family.

Schools again had to be found, Lello and I went to a Presbyterian school, which was a good school and we were there for two years. Violet became a housekeeper and Eve went to college for secretarial training. Father had not yet married and was hoping and trying hard to avoid doing so, but Lily kept a tight hold on him. In addition a broken engagement might have caused a scandal affecting the Irish Church Mission. So at last the marriage could not be put off any longer and the ceremony took place.

That indeed was a dreadful day for us. We all tried to make the best of it, and we prepared a nice meal for the occasion. Later when Father went up to the bedroom, he soon returned with a very anxious look, and said, "Lily has gone," she left a note saying she was going away and might never come back. We all realised that I was scared for they quickly made room for me in a corner. By then it was about 4am and I became very sleepy. The soldiers made as much room for me as possible, and even put a kitbag for me to lean against. I told them that I had to change at Northampton, Peterborough and Ely. They said 'Don't worry, we will wake you in good time for the change'. This they did. it was so kind of them. I was just fifteen and had never been on such a long journey by myself before. I arrived safely at Norwich where my Grandfather was waiting to meet me. I was given such a loving welcome and my Grandmother exclaimed "Where, oh where is my little Rennie?"

I had grown so tall since she had last seen me. I was now 5ft 4ins. This growth was due, I think, to so much cycling and swimming.

I stayed with my Grandparents for five years, for me they were very lonely years. World War I was at its worst phase, food was scarce, and apart from helping to nurse Grandmother, who was now an invalid and only partly mobile, I worked in the garden looking after twenty chickens and some ducks. Life was rather grim. At that time it was for most people for food was rationed and the quality was poor.

Looking back I realise that my time at Norwich was a good training for the future, but I missed mixing with others of my own age group. It certainly taught me to rely on my own resources.

Aunty Lois was very kind to me and tried to make me feel happy and at home, but in spite of her efforts they were lonely years.

I missed the companionship of my sisters and my friend, Edna Bevan.

In such a strict Christian atmosphere, one of the most depressing sounds was the tolling of the death bell for each soldier of our village, which seemed to be almost a personal loss. Grandfather tried to visit every relative and to give them Christian comfort. To add to the general misery and anguish of that time there was the terrible influenza epidemic which was sweeping the whole of Europe.

Grandfather was strict about books, so I had to be careful about what I read. Even the purest of books came under his supervision. I could not read anything other than Christian works, except within a volume of the Biblical Illustrator! That way I could read without comment. Life was not all work or church services; Aunty Lois had a bicycle and I used to go long rides in the country, and sometimes I dared to take a rowing boat and explore the Broads.

Grandfather was Minister to a Non-conformist church, the sermons that he preached were far away above the heads of the people. I remember how persuasive and full of wisdom his homilies were. During this period my Grandmother's health caused a lot of anxiety, she had frequent heart attacks and the doctor was often called to help. On each occasion we thought that she was going to die, the doctor and with Grandfather's earnest prayers between them she would recover. These deathbed scenes occurred for months, and so many of the family would travel quite long distances to say goodbye, and she would have rallied by the time that they had arrived. Though these occasions were trying for all those concerned, they did break into what was rather a dreary time for us. This was about the worst time of the war, the casualties in France were terrible. At times we could hear the guns on the other side of the English Channel. Air raids were becoming more frequent, but nothing like the bombing raids of the second world war, but they were terrifying for single planes would fly low and drop their bombs on farms and factories. I remember watching a German plane flying very low over our garden. Luckily the pilot found nothing worth wasting a bomb on, fortunately for a girl who was hanging out some washing on the line at the time!

Grandmother's heart condition became much worse and she died peacefully in her sleep.

This meant the break up of the home, because Grandfather wanted to live in London near the publishers of his books on the Christian religion. So he and Aunty Lois lived in a London flat, which left me at a loose end. For a time I lived with different relatives, and was really a home help. I hated being dependent.

I was not qualified to do anything except housework and nursing difficult old folk. Eve, my sister, had a friend who was doing her training at King's College Hospital where she was very happy. So I applied and found that Probationers had four hours off every day and two days off a month, when I could do whatever I liked. This after my sheltered life seemed almost too wonderful. When I went for my interview Sister-Matron asked me why I had chosen King's College Hospital. I remember feeling quite embarrassed at this question. I could not say "Because it has the best off duty." So I mumbled something about Denmark Hill was a much nicer place than living in Central London. However I was accepted. The doctor who attended my Grandmother had given me a wonderful recommendation and that was a good start. I must mention that the hospital was 'consecrated', which is why Sister-Matron was so called and the nursing staff had to have their heads covered within the building.

I was told that my uniform would be in my bedroom when I started my training, so I did not stop to try it on before going on to the ward, because I had already been fitted for it. When I tried it on, the dress came down to my feet and I felt awful! There was no time to make it shorter. I had to go on to the men's ward like that.

The men took one look and started to sing, "She's my baby"! Sister let me off early to put a tuck in my dress.

I was very happy at King's and greatly enjoyed my training, the lectures, the nursing and even the cleaning, but most of all the companionship of girls of my own age. We had lots of fun, something I had not had since leaving Ireland. I did not find any of the training too difficult but just lapped it up. When I was sent to the Ear, Nose and Throat department in outpatients I was sorry, because the outpatients were not as interesting as ward patients. However I soon found a great interest in my work.

One day I was preparing the tables with instruments for the different surgeons for examining patients, when the door to the department was very tentatively opened and a rather nervous young man put his head round the door. He was not wearing the usual surgeon's white coat, but one with a most peculiar muddy blue. I went forward to stop this intruder coming any further but he said, "I am a clinical assistant and this is my table."

I thought I would start him off with children and see how he got on with them. He was an instant success, the children were all happy with him and so was I. Little did I think that this shy young man would mean so much to me. He may have been shy, but he certainly had ideas. A few days later I was cleaning instruments in Out Patients when he turned up and asked me whether I had seen a small bottle of chromic acid crystals, which he had inadvertently left. Then he invited me to go to a King's rugger match for the hospital cup. I had to refuse as I had already been invited by one of my friends to go with her to watch the match, and never have I been so bored with such a rough and tumble, and to make matters worse to see King's being soundly beaten in spite of having two international players in the team. I must tell you that as he was talking to me about the match, Home Sister turned up and said in a stern voice, "What do you want, Mr.

Robinson? There is no outpatient session today." Nothing daunted, he replied "I left this bottle of chromic acid crystals last Thursday by mistake." Sister looked very sceptical and I felt embarrassed. However when Sister had gone, he invited me out for a run in his car and to have tea somewhere. I did say yes, and met him at the corner of Caldicote Road with his car. He said, "This is my car" with an expansive wave of his hand. I looked at the car and was not particularly impressed especially as when I sat in the front passenger seat, the back went down, and so did I! The reason this happened was that when he performed minor operations in his surgery at home, he would lift the patient on to the front seat and if necessary let down the back, if the patient could not afford an ambulance. He did not tell me this at the time or I might have had second thoughts about driving with a lunatic! However to proceed with my story, we drove for some time and I recognised where we were and I asked, "Where are we going? He looked a bit guilty and replied 'To the Chiselhurst Caves'. I knew about the Chiselhurst caves and was filled with apprehension. He made a tentative effort to hold my hand, but nothing doing! Poor Geoffrey! I had had a very prim upbringing. The caves were not particularly interesting, we were told that they were prehistoric and dug out by using the horns and shoulder blades of animals. When we came out we had tea at a restaurant and I had my own back by insisting that he be 'Mother' and pour out the tea. (Later the Chiselhurst Caves served a useful purpose during the Second World War as an air raid shelter and also for growing excellent mushrooms. Then back to King's. I enjoyed our little outing and was quite happy to make a date for a future occasion. At that time I was working for my finals, so had to restrict the number of outings with Geoffrey. (Yes we had got as far as Christian names and in 1923 that was rapid progress).

Geoffrey's Mother invited me to tea. She wrote a charming little note to which I immediately replied. When I was introduced to her, I had quite a chilly reception and I wondered why? I eventually found out the reason. Weeks after the tea party Mrs Robinson came up to me and said she was sorry that I had had such a cold reception, but she had not received my letter. One of the maids had put it on the sideboard and it had been covered up. Some weeks later she had dusted the sideboard and my letter was found. (Some maid!)

Now I must tell you about the tea party. All the brothers were there and a young student. I was sitting opposite Oliver. He had a chocolate cake in front of him. He started cutting it and eating it slice after slice, offering it to no one else. When he looked up and saw me watching him consume all the cake except the last piece, he thrust the plate towards me and said, "Would you like some chocolate cake?" Much amused I said "No thank you, please do finish it." Which he promptly did! I forgot to say how charmed I was with Geoffrey's father. He was a delightful man, humorous and kind, and told many stories about his work. He was interested in the fact that I knew the South-West country where he had lived previously, and that I stayed with my Uncle Ben, who was the vicar of a parish near Truro.

After tea Geoffrey's mother regaled us with one of her recitations. She had a wonderful reputation and was in great demand for concerts and entertainments. I had a very happy afternoon. Geoffrey took me back to King's, where I faced a with a barrage of questions, "How had I got on with Geoffrey's family?"

I was warned that our finals were in a few days time. I had already got behind hand with swotting and felt disinclined to get down to start again.

I did get down to study and I passed my finals. I may add with credit, and was then made a State Registered Nurse. This meant much more responsibility, especially when I was given two or sometimes three theatres to run, which meant preparing for operations, putting out the right instruments, catgut and silkworm gut, swabs and dressings. I had to know the number of swabs used internally and count them when the operation was finished.

I remember one occasion, I counted the swabs and one was missing. I counted carefully a second time, still one short, I turned to the surgeon and said, "Sorry, Sir, I am still one short." He felt around and the staff helped, still short, and the surgeon, who was a very impatient busy man, asked me for the sutures. I replied, "Sorry Sir, I cannot give them, until I find the stray one." He got very cross and insisted that I gave them to him. I refused and said, "Why not look again in the abdomen?" He did so and found the missing swab. My relief was great, but there was no apology from the surgeon. However I must say that was the only time that I met such behaviour. Another of my duties was to make sure that all the students' gowns were returned to the dressing room and hung up. This was the rule soon after the 1914 war, as all gowns if they were clean had to be resterilised before use. I looked round and saw that nearly all the gowns were on the floor, and I asked them to "Please pick them up", but they all refused and I said, "All right, you stay there until you pick them up." I walked out locking the door behind me.

Presently the surgeon came out looking for his dressers, not finding them, he asked me where they were. I said "They are locked in the dressing room until they hang up their gowns."

He was furious, but knew that I was right, so he shouted out, "Hang up your gowns!" I then unlocked the door and they came out looking very sheepish. I must add that this was the only time I had any trouble with the dressers.

As I had three operating theatres to run, it was an exhausting job. I was very relieved when the end of my training came. It had been a very happy time for me, and I shall always look back on that period of my life at King's as a most satisfying one.

Now for the next decision! I started my training intending to become a Sister Tutor and to travel to India to train Indian girls. At the same time I had met Geoffrey and had to make up my mind which was it to be - marriage or career? It did not take me long to decide. Marriage won! Geoffrey was on a visit to my Aunt Lois's home, where I was living at the time. We went for a long walk to North Cray village, turned up a road leading to a hill where there were one or two houses. There was an empty cottage standing alone, and it looked as though it was waiting for us. We got the key and found that it was quite a big cottage, two living rooms, kitchen, bathroom, two big and one small bedroom, and all other necessities. This was to be our future home, but where to find the money to run it? Geoffrey would put his plate up and I would help him by being theatre nurse, matron and skivvy.

I left King's on December the 14th, we married on the 19th, had a weekend honeymoon and started married life on a shoestring! The shoe-string lengthened but we were hard up for a long time, but we were confident the we would make a go of it. I have said that the cottage was in a pretty lane which continued up the hill to woods, a turn right brought us to an open field where we had our picnics. This ideal landscape led of course to lots of visitors.

It was rather a strain when I found that I was pregnant. Our first child, Elizabeth, was born on the 14th February 1927. She was a fairy baby, weighing only four and a half pounds, not thin, but just like a live and lovable doll.

We were thrilled with our baby, who was the first baby girl in the Robinson family for two generations. Friends and relatives came to see our wonderful baby and we were very proud parents. She may have given us all joy, but she certainly prevented much progress for the nursing home, however we persevered and just about paid our way.

I have said that our cottage was in a pretty lane and continuing up the hill we came to woods, then a turn right brought us to a field where we had our picnics. That of course meant lots of visitors. One week we had so many visitors that we had no food for Monday morning breakfast!

Geoffrey's father was very ill at this time, and was unable to work. Geoffrey, having no daily surgeries, was called in to take his father's place, which he did for many weeks. Naturally this took time from our small practice, and that suffered as a result. His father did not recover and Geoffrey carried on doing all his work.

His two brothers, Jack and Oliver, between them decided that Geoffrey would be paid £400 a year, and they would divide the rest between themselves until Geoffrey could come in as a full partner and live in the top flat of 186 The Rye, the house where the surgeries were and all messages were taken. This would have meant giving up our cottage and the practice as well as the Ear, Nose and Throat work that Geoffrey was doing. We both felt very deeply over the brothers suggestion and came to the conclusion that we could not give up our lovely little home, and I did not like the idea of Peckham air for my baby. Family ructions started! Geoffrey continued to help in the old practice, but continued working in North Cray.

This all sounds rather complicated, but it worked fairly well, and our small operating theatre was kept quite busy with the two practices.

Although I said there were family ructions, our baby, Elizabeth, was a joy to everyone. The family of Robinsons were all delighted to have such a pretty girl at last born into the family. Five boys had been born to my mother-in-law and her delight was great to have a granddaughter.

When she knew that I was pregnant, she gave me a doll that she had dressed beautifully in the fond hope that it would influence my pregnancy and produce a girl.

Elizabeth remained tiny for a long time, and we were delighted when she bumped her head when running under a table, a thing she did when playing bo-peep.

We had a big garden and grew our own vegetables and lots of flowers. One spring we had lots of daffodils and were very proud of our display. To our dismay one morning we came down and found that they were all gone. The gypsies had taken them!

About this time an elderly doctor who practiced in Bexley had a heart attack and Geoffrey was asked if he would take on his practice. This Geoffrey did and eventually at the doctor's death he was doing all his work. This meant a tremendous increase in his work load, and he found that working from North Cray was too much, so he included the two practices into one and he was asked to take over the house of the doctor.

We were very reluctant to do so as it was very big and quite beyond our means, but eventually we did so and found it a great strain. So I started to take patients in again, both chronically sick and E.N.T. patients for operation. This meant a tremendous lot of extra work and I had to have help.

I became pregnant again and our second daughter, Patricia, was born on the 27th October 1928. I went to a nursing home for her birth. The matron had done a lot of work for Geoffrey and she reduced the fees for Patricia. She was a bonny baby and when I took her in my arms I found that the umbilical cord had not been tied off properly, and she was losing quite a lot of blood. I called to matron, who sent for the doctor and between them they stopped the bleeding. I was very scared and refused to let matron take the baby from me but held her in my arms all night to give her my body warmth. She recovered all right but it did pull her down for some time. However she was soon well back to being a bonny baby. Patricia was such a contented and happy baby and gave us no further trouble or anxiety. Two babies and one or two patients meant a great deal of work and I continued to need help. I advertised and got quite a good nurse and together we made a fair success of our home. The house was called Grangehurst and was charming with a lovely garden including a tennis court, huge vegetable garden and many fruit trees. We could have been happy there but the strain was too much. I was ill for a time but made a quick recovery. Then Geoffrey was out on a night call, got drenched by a downpour, and a bad cold developed into rheumatic fever. He was ill for over a year. Oliver helped with the practice, while I tried to keep things going but found it almost impossible. We eventually moved into our surgery, which was a charming old house about 250 years old, very convenient for the patients and for the doctor but we were cramped for room. The practice grew rapidly, and we felt that we would soon be in a position to have a larger house. A house became vacant in Parkhurst Road large enough to have a surgery and waiting room. It had five bedrooms and good domestic arrangements. So we decided to buy it.

It seemed that our worries were at an end. The house was ideal for the practice, a good garden for the children to play in and a school nearby.

I became pregnant again, and on the 23rd April 1934 Waring was born; just what we wanted to complete our family. He was a lovely baby, very fair, weighing eight and three quarter pounds, and our happiness seemed complete. The practice was doing well and Geoffrey was a surgeon at the Children's Hospital at Sydendam.

War clouds were looming ahead and Germany was again our enemy. A truly awful man, Adolf Hitler, became ruler in Germany, and he was determined to control Europe. Our prime minister went to Germany almost to intercede, he came back with a signed piece of paper which would give peace in our time. That peace lasted about a year, then Hitler started his venomous war. That year did give us a little time to prepare for all the horror that Germany could throw at us. The bombing did not start until about a year after that. In the meantime we made our preparations which beside German preparations were insignificant. Geoffrey's and my preparations were to have another child. Morris was born on twenty eighth of March, just nine months before the Second World War started.

You could not fine a happier baby than Morris. He was so content and if anyone looked at him he would give a big smile. I remember later on I had to return to London, when we were evacuated during the early part of the war, in order to check our furniture. I could not take all the family but only Morris and the train was crowded. A man pushed his way into our carriage, but got out again only to return immediately.

He said, "No room anywhere so I came back to the baby carriage." He smiled at Morris and was awarded with a happy grin! He then began to chat and said, "I didn't want a crying baby." In fact they got on fine. Morris was the happiest baby a mother could have, and he was sunshine all the way. He was born before the war but he always brought peace. Geoffrey was on the reserve because he had been in the First World War. His dilemma was should he join up again or stay at home to run a big practice? There were two other doctors in Bexley, both Irish and neither would join up. The first man had been a missionary and felt that war was the wrong way to settle differences, and the second doctor was not expected to live long.

We lived in Bexley about twelve miles from London and we knew that we would be in the direct line for bombing, so we decided to pack up as much as we could of our possessions and placed them in the cellar and locked the door.

The we made tracks for Bristol where we had some friends. They were the Rudolf family. Gerald was Geoffrey's friend. Gerald's father was the founder of the Church of England's 'Waifs and Strays Society' which had a wonderful name in the 'Charities'. They found a place for us to put our caravan, and we prepared for the night.

It was a strange and anxious time. Geoffrey had to go back to a lonely and empty house, and he did more preparations for expected air raids. He received his call up papers and went to a tailor in Bristol for his uniform. In the meantime I made arrangements with Rosemary Rudolf to share her home and between us turned her bungalow into an air raid shelter for eight children and three women because my sister Eva and her three girls joined us too. It is so quick and easy to write about but to organise was a long and exhausting job.

Meanwhile Geoffrey was sent to northern France and preparations were made to push the Germans back and to train the army for the onslaught which we knew was coming. It was not long before the real war started and we were forced to retreat. The fighting was heavy and bitter but the army was pushed back and the now famous retreat ended with many of our men being taken prisoners.

Geoffrey managed to find a boat and got as many men as he could on to it. It was a flat bottomed boat however and very slow; it had one good point, it floated high over the mines!. I wish I could give the number of men who got away, but there were enough to start the army again.

Geoffrey was appointed E.N.T. surgeon at Colchester Military Hospital where he worked for a year before being sent to West Africa. On the whole he enjoyed his time in the Gambia, and quite enjoyed working with the Gambians in the hospital. He certainly had experience of tropical diseases, which he could not have had if he remained in England. He stayed there for nearly two years.

We were enduring the most appalling air raids and much of London was flat, and Bristol, near where we were staying was largely destroyed. I will not dwell on all the horrors of air warfare, except to say that I decided to return to Bexley. The bombing had increased in Bristol so much that I felt the risk was equal in Bristol or London, and we had excellent cellars in Bexley. We collected all our belongings and once again went back to our home. I immediately prepared our cellars for living and sleeping in and we had an air raid shelter fixed up. This was made of thick steel on top and bottom with strong steel mesh sides. We got in and out by crawling one after another. The four children and I managed with great difficulty to get in but we managed every time. The children complained about the nearest breathing on them. I was very firm about the cat sharing our shelter, the children wanted it to sleep with us but I said, "No, cats smell and I cannot stand it." I put her in the corner and said she could sleep there.

Nights became nightmares, and I wondered so often if we would survive. We did survive for a short time until a flying bomb landed in the garden and we were badly shaken. Windows were broken and furniture thrown about and part of the roof fell in. We had to move so I rang my uncle living in Westmoreland and he said "Come at once!" So once again we left our ruined house. Unfortunately Elizabeth and I could not travel with the children because she had to take her examination. I took the children to Euston and found it crowded with parents and children. While we were waiting for the train the air raid warning sounded and we quickly got onto the train. I had a hasty goodbye to the three children. Waring thought that he would cheer us up by saying,

"Never mind Mummy, if you get killed Daddy will still have us." This caused a general laugh in the carriage and the gloom was lifted for a short time. Elizabeth and I returned to Bexley and the next day Elizabeth started her examinations which took about five days.

I am happy to report that she passed well. She and I then went to Kendal, and my aunt and uncle managed to make room for five of us in their small house. The scenery was lovely and the nights peaceful. The girls continued their education by doing an Oxford correspondence course. Waring I sent to a school in Kendal.

The peace was wonderful for a time and our fears were allayed and most of my anxiety was for Geoffrey. He was still in West Africa and on the whole enjoyed the experience. The Gambians were very superstitious and feared all sorts of horrors. Geoffrey was made second in command of the hospital and came home after two years. He arrived late at night while the children were in bed fast asleep. In the morning Morris, who was sleeping on a camp bed in my room, took one look at his sleeping father, and shouted, "Who is that man sleeping in your bed?" When I explained who the strange man was he jumped into bed and gave the strange man a big hug. We were a family again. It was some time before Geoffrey was officially retired from the army and we could consider getting our home together again. We were given a small three bedroom house, and then went to the hall where the remains of our furniture were stored. We were horrified at the condition of most of it. Our ladder back dining room chairs had been thrown about and weakened. However with Uncle Finn's help we got them more or less repaired and usable again.

It was a very uphill job starting again, and many of our patients had left the district because of the war. The girls started again at their old school, Babington House School at Eltham, but they were not happy there. Elizabeth had taken and passed her matriculation. She wanted to read medicine. She applied and was told that she would have to wait some years. There were so many men who had been in the services, who hoped to do the same, that the girls had to wait. As she was most disappointed, she decided to do the next best thing in the medical field and started her training as a radiographer. She completed her training easily and was soon rewarded with a post in a hospital at Dartford.

Paddy finished her schooling and decided to train as a nurse. She started her training at Great Ormond Street Hospital just as we moved to Leicester. Ill health forced her to stop nursing and she surprised us all by saying she wanted to go on the stage. A shyer more unobstrusive girl could not be found, but if that was what she wanted, we would see what could be done. Geoffrey made an appointment with a senior person at R.A.D.A. who gave him advice how Paddy should train. She eventually went to the Birmingham School of Speech Training and Dramatic Art. It had a good name, but I felt it was the wrong thing for Paddy. She had great skill in the arts but not in performance. Her painting and drawing were good and she had particular skill in clothes design and in the use of materials, she was also good at life drawing, but she was always looking for something different.

Whilst at the Birmingham School of Speech Training and Dramatic Art she met and became engaged to one of the most gifted students. He was a very talented actor, but we were not at all happy about the engagement. Paddy married John and followed him soon after he went to New York. She wished to work with young children, but found that she was not sufficiently trained, so she enrolled at the City College of New York and trained as a teacher. The marriage ended and Paddy made a new life for herself in California and eventually settled in San Francisco, and has remained in that lovely city ever since. I hope Paddy will tell the story of her own life in the U.S.A. and how she succeeded there.

Geoffrey had obtained an important specialist post in Leicester, where we now made our home. Waring and Morris went to school. Waring to Oundle, and Morris to a prep school. After a year in Leicester we moved to a thatched cottage in the village of Billesdon and had a very happy three years there. At times with all the children with us there we became involved in all aspects of village life.

Sadly the changes brought about by the National Health Service reduced Geoffrey's income and we decided to move back to Leicester partly to reduce his travelling and partly to share a house with my sister, Eva, following the death of her husband, Sidney. We stayed there until Geoffrey retired in 1961.

In the meantime as already mentioned, Paddy had married and gone to the United States and Elizabeth had married a very talented painter, Kenneth Hill. Before we left Leicester, Ken painted Geoffrey's portrait, which was accepted and shown at the Summer exhibition at the Royal Academy.

Waring completed his schooling, then had to do his National Service before he could start his medical training at St. George's Hospital. Morris went to Bloxham School, and then to Leicester University to study for Social Work. He finished there at the same time that Geoffrey retired and Morris then started work in Birmingham.

Now began one of the happiest times of our lives. In 1959 we had bought a plot of land near Bude in Cornwall. My sister, Eva, had settled in the village a little earlier, so as to be near her daughter,

Biddy, and her family. Geoffrey's brother, Jack, lived at Lostwithiel so there were several links with Cornwall. We had some expert help, but we did most of the work ourselves in erecting a cedar wood bungalow, and all the work in creating a garden. We had a large orchard, where the experts said none of the trees would grow, and there were wonderful views over sweeping headlands to the Atlantic.

This home proved to be a very special place for us to welcome our visiting family and it is a great joy that six of our grandchildren will always have memories of Moorcroft, Poughill. Meanwhile Waring completed his medical studies and started to practice as a General Practitioner in Hertford, but not before he had been the mainstay in building Moorcroft. There was underfloor heating, which we covered with parquet. It was a very warm bungalow. The living room was L-shaped, the long part was the sitting room and the small part the dining area. This took our table and chairs and dresser with a large window overlooking the front garden. The sitting room had an even larger window from which we could enjoy our developing garden and the wide vista of the Cornish coast. There were two double bedrooms. Moving in was one of the happiest days of our lives. The furniture fitted in so well, and we had plenty of cupboard space. We were so happy and although we worked hard in the garden, the result was worth the labour.

I have described the building in detail because it was the perfect bungalow for our retirement. Geoffrey had great ideas for the garden. He decided to make it a paying proposition, and so planned to plant 200 apple trees (George Cave, Russets, and Worcesters). These were all a success and we sold them to visitors to Cornwall. Our coastline was very attractive, rocky and sandy where children could play with safety in the pools, and older visitors had a lovely time surfing in the Atlantic breakers. Altogether it was a wonderful home, and we could not have been happier. We found retirement was expensive which led Geoffrey to undertake various locum posts particularly in Northern Ireland and Pontypool. It was stimulating to go somewhere else, but so exciting and rewarding to return to our Cornish dream home.

Geoffrey was ill twice and gave us both a fright, but each time it proved to be nothing serious. You will wonder why did we leave after thirteen years? I will not go into the whys and wherefores, enough to say that I did not want to leave, but circumstances made it impossible to stay. Waring was extending his bungalow and decided to include a flat for us. Of course this meant that we would see more of the family, and Morris and Barbara had moved to Oxfordshire only two hours from Waring and Alison. London was only a short distance from Hertford which meant we could go up to the theatre occasionally.

We settled down. But year after year passed by, and I came to feel that we ought to leave Waring and Alison to their own home and suggested very often that we found somewhere else. Whenever I suggested a move Geoffrey would reply, "Waring said that we could stay here until we died." Unfortunately we failed to die and our few years extended to eighteen. They had had enough and we knew it was right to move on, and that we could no longer manage on our own, even though we had been looking after ourselves with the minimum of help.

We celebrated our Golden and Diamond wedding anniversaries at the Pightle. Morris hunted around in Oxfordshire for a retirement home and so in July 1992 we came to Newland House in Witney. We are very comfortable for the most part but it seems very expensive, and our capital has been whittled down. I understand that we now have some regular financial help to keep us going.

We are very old, Geoffrey is 97 and I will soon be 94! Why are we living so long? I am coming to the end of our life story, as I am sure we are near the end, and I feel that I want to leave some farewell thoughts to you all, and Geoffrey joins me in this, but he is writing his own memoirs.

I am sure that he has much to say writing his own life story.

You have been a wonderful family to have, faults and all. I hope that you will be happy and helpful to one another. To our grandchildren and great-grandchildren, may your futures be as good and fulfilling as your dreams of the future are. You all seem to be choosing good and sound professions, or doing well at school or university.

God bless you all.